A Human Health Perspective On Climate Change

A Report Outlining the Research Needs on the Human Health Effects of Climate Change

Published by
Environmental Health Perspectives and
the National Institute of
Environmental Health Sciences

A Human Health Perspective
On Climate Change

A Report Outlining the Research Needs on the Human Health Effects of Climate Change

The Interagency Working Group on Climate Change and Health[1] (IWGCCH)

1   DISCLAIMER: The Interagency Working Group on Climate Change and Health (IWGCCH) is an ad hoc group formed by participating federal agencies and organizations at the invitation of the National Institute of Environmental Health Sciences (NIEHS), National Oceanic and Atmospheric Administration (NOAA), Centers for Disease Control and Prevention (CDC), and Environmental Protection Agency (EPA) following the January 2009 "Workshop on a Research Agenda for Managing the Health Risks of Climate Change," sponsored by the Institute of Medicine Roundtable on Environmental Health Sciences, Research, and Medicine. This report identifies gaps in knowledge of the consequences for human health of climate change, and suggests research to address them. The content, views, and perspectives presented in this report are solely those of the authors, and do not reflect the official views, policies, or implied endorsement of any of the individual participating federal agencies or organizations.

Published by Environmental Health Perspectives and the National Institute of Environmental Health Sciences

Environmental Health Perspectives (ISSN 0091-6765) is a peer-reviewed publication of the Public Health Service, U.S. Department of Health and Human Services. *EHP* is an open-access monthly journal of peer-reviewed research and news on the impact of the environment on human health. *EHP* also publishes a quarterly *Chinese Edition* (ISSN 1542-6351) and occasional special issues. The Secretary of Health and Human Services has deemed *EHP* to be necessary in the transaction of the public business required by law of this department.

CORRESPONDENCE: Send all correspondence to Hugh A. Tilson, PhD, Editor-In-Chief, *EHP*, NIEHS/NIH, Mail Drop K3-01, PO Box 12233, Research Triangle Park, NC 27709 USA; phone: 919-541-3280; e-mail: EHPEditor@niehs.nih.gov.

COPYRIGHT, REPRODUCTION, AND CITATION: *EHP* is a publication of the U.S. government. Publication of *EHP* lies in the public domain and is therefore without copyright. Research and News articles from *EHP* may be reprinted freely; however, News articles may contain photographs or figures copyrighted by commercial organizations or individuals that may not be used without obtaining prior approval from the holder of the copyright. Use of materials published in *EHP* should be acknowledged (for example, "Reproduced with permission from *Environmental Health Perspectives* "), and pertinent reference information should be provided for the article from which the material was reproduced. For further information, contact *EHP* Permissions (ehponline@niehs.nih.gov).

DISCLAIMER: The publication of articles and advertising in this journal does not mean that the National Institute of Environmental Health Sciences (NIEHS) condones, endorses, approves, or recommends the use of any products, services, materials, methodology, or policies stated therein. Conclusions and opinions are those of the individual authors and advertisers only and do not reflect the policies or views of the NIEHS.

DISCRIMINATION PROHIBITED: Under the provisions of applicable public laws enacted by Congress since 1964, no person in the United States shall, on the grounds of race, color, national origin, handicap, or age, be excluded from participation in, be denied the benefits of, or be subjected to discrimination under any program or activity (or, on the basis of sex, with respect to any educational program or activity) receiving Federal financial assistance. In addition, Executive Order 11141 prohibits discrimination on the basis of age by contractors and subcontractors in the performance of Federal contracts, and Executive Order 11246 states that no federally funded contractor may discriminate against any employee or applicant for employment because of race, color, religion, sex, or national origin. Therefore, the NIEHS must be operated in compliance with these laws and executive orders.

Table of Contents

The Interagency Working Group on Climate Change and Health

Christopher J. Portier, PhD (COORDINATING LEAD AUTHOR)
National Institute of Environmental Health Sciences

Kimberly Thigpen Tart, JD (COORDINATING EDITOR)
National Institute of Environmental Health Sciences

Sarah R. Carter, PhD
AAAS Fellow, U.S. Environmental Protection Agency

Caroline H. Dilworth, PhD
National Institute of Environmental Health Sciences

Anne E. Grambsch
U.S. Environmental Protection Agency

Julia Golke, PhD
National Institute of Environmental Health Sciences

Jeremy Hess, MD, MPH (LEAD AUTHOR)
Centers for Disease Control and Prevention

Sandra N. Howard, PhD
Department of Health and Human Services

George Luber, PhD (LEAD AUTHOR)
Centers for Disease Control and Prevention

Jeffrey T. Lutz, PhD
National Oceanic and Atmospheric Administration

Tanya Maslak, MPH (LEAD AUTHOR)
*U.S. Global Change Research Program,
University Corporation for Atmospheric Research*

Natasha Prudent, MPH
Centers for Disease Control and Prevention

Meghan Radtke, PhD (LEAD AUTHOR)
AAAS Fellow, U.S. Environmental Protection Agency

Joshua P. Rosenthal, PhD
Fogarty International Center

Teri Rowles, DVM, PhD
National Oceanic and Atmospheric Administration

Paul A. Sandifer, PhD
National Oceanic and Atmospheric Administration

Joel Scheraga, PhD
U.S. Environmental Protection Agency

Paul J. Schramm, MS, MPH
Centers for Disease Control and Prevention

Daniel Strickman, PhD (LEAD AUTHOR)
U.S. Department of Agriculture, Agricultural Research Service

Juli M. Trtanj, MES (LEAD AUTHOR)
National Oceanic and Atmospheric Administration

Pai-Yei Whung, PhD
U.S. Environmental Protection Agency

Participating Agencies

In addition to the working group, many scientists and staff from the following agencies contributed to the development and review of this white paper. Staff of the U.S. Global Change Research Program provided logistical and technical support, but did not conduct a formal review.

Centers for Disease Control and Prevention

- National Center for Environmental Health

National Institutes of Health

- National Institute of Environmental Health Sciences
- Fogarty International Center
- Trans-NIH Working Group on Climate Change and Health

National Oceanic and Atmospheric Administration

Office of the Secretary, Department of Health and Human Services

U.S. Environmental Protection Agency

U.S. Department of Agriculture

U.S. Department of State

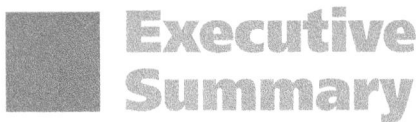

Executive Summary

The purpose of this paper is to identify research needs for all aspects of the research-to-decision making pathway that will help us understand and mitigate the health effects of climate change, as well as ensure that we choose the healthiest and most efficient approaches to climate change adaptation.

Climate change endangers human health, affecting all sectors of society, both domestically and globally. The environmental consequences of climate change, both those already observed and those that are anticipated, such as sea-level rise, changes in precipitation resulting in flooding and drought, heat waves, more intense hurricanes and storms, and degraded air quality, will affect human health both directly and indirectly. Addressing the effects of climate change on human health is especially challenging because both the surrounding environment and the decisions that people make influence health. For example, increases in the frequency and severity of regional heat waves—likely outcomes of climate change—have the potential to harm a lot of people. Certain adverse health effects can probably be avoided if decisions made prior to the heat waves result in such things as identification of vulnerable populations such as children and the elderly and ensured access to preventive measures such as air conditioning. This is a simplified illustration; in real-life situations a host of other factors also come into play in determining vulnerability including biological susceptibility, socioeconomic status, cultural competence, and the built environment. In a world of myriad "what if" scenarios surrounding climate change, it becomes very complicated to create wise health policies for the future because of the uncertainty of predicting environmental change and human decisions. The need for sound science on which to base such policies becomes more critical than ever.

Recognizing the complexity of this issue, an ad hoc Interagency Working Group on Climate Change and Health (IWGCCH)[2] assembled to develop a white paper on relevant federal research and science needs, including research on mitigation and adaptation strategies. Examples of mitigation and adaptation research needs are identified, but a comprehensive discussion of these issues is not included. These research and science needs broadly include basic and applied science, technological innovations and capacities, public health infrastructure, and communication and education. Consideration is also given to the potential structure of a federal climate change and health research agenda and the use of scientific research results for applications and decision making. The purpose of this paper is to identify research critical for understanding the impact of climate change on human health so that we can both mitigate and adapt to the environmental effects of climate change in the healthiest and most efficient ways. Although the group recognizes the global nature of climate change's impacts on human health, the primary focus of this paper is on the situation in the United States.

This report is organized around 11 broad human health categories likely to be affected by climate change.[3] Categories are arranged in alphabetical order, and no prioritization—for instance as to likelihood of occurrence, severity of effects, or depth of current knowledge—is implied. Each category is broken into sections that introduce the topic, explain its

relationship to climate change, and identify the basic and applied research needs of that category, as well as crosscutting issues where relevant. Most investigations of climate change and health have relied on environmental and ecological effects to extrapolate potential human health impacts; the IWGCCH deliberately chose to emphasize the need for research on human health outcomes over environmental impacts for this reason: this approach highlights direct links between climate change and federal research priorities that are often disease- or outcome-specific, and a focus on human health outcomes enables a holistic approach to exploring climate change-related health impacts. We recognize that the health consequences identified in this document are not exhaustive, and that because so many climate change effects are prospective, some of the research needs enumerated may be speculative. As more information becomes available, new research needs may be identified and others rejected, but it is our intent that this report may serve as a baseline discussion from which agencies can proceed.

---

2   CDC, HHS/OS, EPA, NASA, NIEHS, NIH/Fogarty, NOAA, DOS, USDA, USGCRP
3   asthma, allergies, and airway diseases; cancer; cardiovascular disease and stroke; alterations in normal development; heat-related morbidity and mortality; mental health and stress disorders; neurological diseases and disorders; nutrition and food-borne illness; vector-borne and zoonotic disease; waterborne disease; weather-related morbidity and mortality

Highlights:

Asthma, Respiratory Allergies, and Airway Diseases—
Respiratory allergies and diseases may become more prevalent because of increased human exposure to pollen (due to altered growing seasons), molds (from extreme or more frequent precipitation), air pollution and aerosolized marine toxins (due to increased temperature, coastal runoff, and humidity) and dust (from droughts). Mitigation and adaptation may significantly reduce these risks. Research should address the relationship between climate change and the composition of air pollutant mixtures (e.g., how altered pollen counts and other effects of climate change affect the severity of asthma) to produce models to identify populations at risk. Such tools support the use of science in understanding disease risks and as such, are an integral component of developing effective risk communication and targeting the messages to vulnerable populations.

Cancer—Many potential direct effects of climate change on cancer risk, such as increased duration and intensity of ultraviolet (UV) radiation, are well understood; however the potential impact of changes in climate on exposure pathways for chemicals and toxins requires further study. Science should investigate the effects of mitigation and adaptation measures on cancer incidence so that the best strategies can be developed and implemented; for example, research to inform understanding of the benefits of alternative fuels, new battery and voltaic cells, and other technologies, as well as any potential adverse risks from exposure to their components and wastes. Better understanding of climate change impacts on the capacity of ocean and coastal systems to provide cancer curative agents and other health-enhancing products is also needed.

Cardiovascular Disease and Stroke—Climate change may exacerbate existing cardiovascular disease by increasing heat stress, increasing the body burden of airborne particulates, and changing the distribution of zoonotic vectors that cause infectious diseases linked with cardiovascular disease. Science that addresses the cardiovascular effects of higher temperatures, heat waves, extreme weather, and changes in air quality on health is needed, and this new information should be applied to development of health risk assessment models, early warning systems, health communication strategies targeting vulnerable populations, land use decisions, and strategies to meet air quality goals related to climate change. In some areas, cardiovascular and stroke risks resulting from climate change could be offset by reductions in air pollution due to climate change mitigation.

Foodborne Diseases and Nutrition—Climate change may be associated with staple food shortages, malnutrition, and food contamination (of seafood from chemical contaminants, biotoxins, and pathogenic microbes, and of crops by pesticides). Science research needs in this area include better understanding of how changes in agriculture and fisheries may affect food availability and nutrition, better monitoring for disease-causing agents, and identification and mapping of complex food webs and sentinel species that may be vulnerable to climate change. This research could be used to prepare the public health and health care sectors for new illnesses, changing surveillance needs, and increased incidence of disease, as well as development of more effective outreach to affected communities.

Heat-Related Morbidity and Mortality—Heat-related illness and deaths are likely to increase in response to climate change but aggressive public health interventions such as heat wave response plans and health alert warning systems can minimize morbidity and mortality. Additional science should be focused on developing and expanding these tools in different geographic regions, specifically by defining environmental risk factors, identifying vulnerable populations, and developing effective risk communication and prevention strategies.

Human Developmental Effects—Two potential consequences of climate change would affect normal human development: malnutrition—particularly during the prenatal period and early childhood as a result of decreased food supplies, and exposure to toxic contaminants and biotoxins—resulting from extreme weather events, increased pesticide use for food production, and increases in harmful algal blooms in recreational areas. Research should examine the relationship between human development and adaptations to climate change, such as agriculture and fisheries changes that may affect food availability, increased pesticide use to control for expanding disease vector ranges, and prevention of leaching from toxic waste sites into floodwaters during extreme weather events, so that developmental consequences can be prevented.

Mental Health and Stress-Related Disorders—By causing or contributing to extreme weather events, climate change may result in geographic displacement of populations, damage to property, loss of loved ones, and chronic stress, all of which can negatively affect mental health. Research needs include identifying key mental health effects and vulnerable populations, and developing migration monitoring networks to help ensure the availability of appropriate health care support.

Neurological Diseases and Disorders—Climate change, as well as attempts to mitigate and adapt to it, may increase the number of neurological diseases and disorders in humans. Research in this area should focus on identifying vulnerable populations and understanding the mechanisms and effects of human exposure to neurological hazards such as biotoxins (from harmful algal blooms), metals (found in new battery technologies and compact fluorescent lights), and pesticides (used in response to changes in agriculture), as well as the potentially exacerbating effects of malnutrition and stress.

Vectorborne and Zoonotic Diseases—Disease risk may increase as a result of climate change due to related expansions in vector ranges, shortening of pathogen incubation periods, and disruption and relocation of large human populations. Research should enhance the existing pathogen/vector control infrastructure including vector and host identification; integrate human with terrestrial and aquatic animal health surveillance systems; incorporate ecological studies to provide better predictive models; and improve risk communication and prevention strategies.

Waterborne Diseases—Increases in water temperature, precipitation frequency and severity, evaporation-transpiration rates, and changes in coastal ecosystem health could increase the incidence of water contamination with harmful pathogens and chemicals, resulting in increased human exposure. Research should focus on understanding where changes in water flow will occur, how water will interact with sewage in surface and underground water supplies as well as drinking water distribution systems, what food sources may become contaminated, and how to better predict and prevent human exposure to waterborne and ocean-related pathogens and biotoxins.

Weather-Related Morbidity and Mortality—Increases in the incidence and intensity of extreme weather events such as hurricanes, floods, droughts, and wildfires may adversely affect people's health immediately during the event or later following the event. Research aimed at improving the capabilities of healthcare and emergency services to address disaster planning and management is needed to ensure that risks are understood and that optimal strategies are identified, communicated, and implemented.

In addition to the research needs identified in the individual research categories, there are crosscutting issues relevant to preventing or avoiding many of the potential health impacts of climate change including identifying susceptible, vulnerable, and displaced populations; enhancing public health and health care infrastructure; developing capacities and skills in modeling and prediction; and improving risk communication and public health education. Such research will lead to more effective early warning systems and greater public awareness of an individual's or community's health risk from climate change, which should translate into more successful mitigation and adaptation

strategies. For example, health communications research is needed to properly implement health alert warning systems for extreme heat events and air pollution that especially affects people with existing conditions such as cardiovascular disease. Such a risk communication pilot project might demonstrate communication practices that are effective in multiple areas, and contribute to a comprehensive strategy for addressing multiple health risks simultaneously.

Other tools are needed and should be applied across multiple categories to close the knowledge gaps, including predictive models to improve forecasting and prevention, evaluations of the vulnerability of health care and public health systems and infrastructure, and health impact assessments. Trans-disciplinary development would help to ensure tools such as improved baseline monitoring that will be more widely applicable, and thus more efficient and cost effective than those currently available. In fact, many of the identified science needs will require trans-disciplinary responses. For example, to study how heat waves alter ambient air pollution and the resulting combined impact of heat and pollution on human illness and death, will require expertise in atmospheric chemistry, climate patterns, environmental health, epidemiology, medicine, and other science fields. Given the complexity of the science needs and the potential overlap of research questions across disciplines, promoting trans-disciplinary collaboration among and within federal agencies would be a logical approach and should be a high priority.

Recently, the National Research Council issued a report addressing how federal research and science could be improved to provide support for decision and policy making on climate change and human health.[4] Specifically, the report calls for a more complete catalogue of climate change health impacts, increasing the power of prediction tools, enhancing integration of climate observation networks with health impact surveillance tools, and improving interactions among stakeholders and decision makers. The IWGCCH approached this research needs assessment with these goals in mind. The next step will be for federal agencies to discuss the findings of this white paper with stakeholders, decision makers, and the public as they work to incorporate and prioritize appropriate research needs into their respective science agendas and collaborative research efforts. A coordinated federal approach will bring the unique skills, capacities, and missions of the various agencies together to maximize the potential for discovery of new information and opportunities for success in providing key information to support responsive and effective decisions on climate change and health.

4   National Research Council (U.S.). Committee on Strategic Advice on the U.S. Climate Change Science Program., et al. 2009, Washington, D.C.: National Academies Press. xii, 254 p.

Introduction

Global climate change has become one of the most visible environmental concerns of the 21st century. From pictures of polar bears clinging to melting ice floes in Alaska to dried and cracked farmland stretching into the horizon in Africa, images of the ecological impacts of climate change have become part of our combined consciousness and inspire concern and discussion about what climate change ultimately will mean to our planet. But seldom are the effects of climate change expressed, either visually or otherwise, in terms of the real and potential costs in human lives and suffering. To date, most climate change research has focused on environmental effects and not health effects. It is clear that climate change endangers human health, but there is need to improve the science and knowledge base of how it occurs. One purpose of this document is to identify research gaps to increase the understanding of climate change and health. Expanding our understanding of the often indirect, long-term, and complex consequences of climate change for human health is a high priority and challenging research task.[5] In the developed world particularly, there is perhaps a greater perception of the ecological and environmental effects of climate change than of the human health implications. This may be due in part to the fact that images linking climate change and some already apparent wildlife and landscape effects are prevalent, and thereby, increase concern.

5   National Research Council (U.S.). Committee On Health, E, And Other External Costs And, et al. Board on Environmental Studies and Toxicology special report. 2009, Washington, D.C.: Board on Environmental Studies and Toxicology.

There is no doubt, however, that climate change is currently affecting public health through myriad environmental consequences, such as sea-level rise, changes in precipitation resulting in flooding and drought, heat waves, changes in intensity of hurricanes and storms, and degraded air quality, that are anticipated to continue into the foreseeable future. In a tally that included just four diseases (cardiovascular disease, malnutrition, diarrhea, and malaria) as well as floods, the World Health Organization (WHO) estimated 166,000 deaths and about 5.5 million disability-adjusted life years (DALYs, a measure of overall disease burden) were attributable to climate change in 2000.[6] To date, the majority of analyses on climate change and health have focused on diseases that predominantly affect people in the developing world, and therefore, are perceived as less relevant to more developed countries. However, as the recent pandemic of H1N1 virus has shown us, diseases do not respect international boundaries. Climate change can be a driver for disease migration, but even so, such diseases do not represent the broadest range of possible, or even likely, human health effects of climate change, nor do they reflect the likely co-benefits of mitigation and adaptation to climate change, some of which may have their greatest impact in the developed world.

For over 170 years, scientists have studied the complicated relationship between the weather, climate, and human health.[7] Since the first attempt at scientific consensus on climate change nearly four decades ago,[8] scientists have been examining whether climate is indeed changing as a result of human activity. However, the complicated relationships between climate change, the environment, and human health have not represented high priorities for scientific research in the United States, and there are abundant gaps in our understanding of these links.[9] Such gaps impair our ability to identify optimal strategies for mitigation and adaptation that will prevent illness and death in current human populations while simultaneously protecting the environment and health of future generations. The purpose of this report is to identify the major research areas that need to be further explored and understood, and to identify the scientific capacities that will be needed to adequately address the problems that arise at the nexus of climate, environment, and human health with the goal of informing federal agencies with a human health or related research mission as they approach these daunting challenges.[10] Research outcomes generated from the needs agenda outlined here would go a

long way toward informing health decision making and addressing the challenges outlined in the National Research Council's report.[11].

Leaders including the Director, National Institute of Environmental Health Sciences (NIEHS); the Chief Scientist in the Office of the Science Advisor, U.S. Environmental Protection Agency (EPA); the Senior Scientist for Coastal Ecology, National Oceanic and Atmospheric Administration (NOAA); and the Director, National Center for Environmental Health, Centers for Disease Control and Prevention (CDC) initiated the development of this white paper in February 2009. The Interagency Working Group on Climate Change and Health (IWGCCH) was established with representation and participation from various federal agencies, institutes, and other organizations with an environmental health or public health mandate. (Participating groups are listed on the Working Group page of this document, pp. iii). The first activity of this ad hoc group was to review and distill the state of the science on the effects of climate change on human health from the many excellent reviews of climate change already published by groups including the Intergovernmental Panel on Climate Change, the World Health Organization, the U.S. Global Change Research Program, the National Research Council, and others. Most of these reports take a much broader view of the issue of climate change; however, the portions that are directly relevant to human health effects provided a critical baseline from which this working group could proceed to identify the research gaps and needs in this area.

This document does not attempt to be a comprehensive assessment of the risks associated with climate change and health or a strategic plan. Rather it seeks to build on the existing knowledge of the prior efforts, and extend this knowledge further by shifting the perspective on climate change effects from a largely ecological and meteorological base to one that focuses on the human health consequences of climate change, mitigation, and adaptation. Similarly, an aim of this report is to inform the federal government as it seeks to focus climate change research on understanding the interactions among the climate, human, and environmental systems and on supporting societal responses to climate change. In this way, it is responsive to the recommendations of some of these reports. The working group has drafted this document in consultation with subject matter experts at the various agencies, seeking their review and comment throughout the process to provide a concise, credible, and broad discussion.

6   Campbell-Lendrum, D, et al. Environmental Burden of Disease Series, ed. A Pruss-Ustun, et al. 2007, Geneva: World Health Organization. 66.

7   Dunglison, R. 1835, Philadelphia,: Carey, Lea & Blanchard. xi, [13]-514 p.

8   Study of Critical Environmental Problems., et al. 1970, Cambridge, Mass.,: MIT Press. xxii, 319 p.

9   Campbell-Lendrum, D, et al., The Lancet, 2009. 373(9676): p. 1663-1665.

10   Gamble, JL, et al. 2008, Washington, D.C.: U.S. Climate Change Science Program. ix, 204 p.

11   National Research Council (U.S.). Committee on Strategic Advice on the U.S. Climate Change Science Program., et al. 2009, Washington, D.C.: National Academies Press. xii, 254 p.

Figure 1 provides the conceptual framework used to develop this report. In addition to the direct effects of heat on humans, the major impacts of climate change on human health are through changes to the human environment such as rising oceans, changing weather patterns, and decreased availability of fresh water. Mitigation of climate change refers to actions being taken to reduce greenhouse gas emissions and to enhance the sinks that trap or remove carbon from the atmosphere to reduce the extent of global climate change. Adaptation refers to actions being taken to lessen the impact on health and the environment due to changes that cannot be prevented through mitigation. Appropriate mitigation and adaptation strategies will positively affect both climate change and the environment, and thereby positively affect human health. In addition, some adaptation activities will directly improve human health through changes in our public health and health care infrastructure. Gaps in our under-standing of how human health, climate change, the environment, and mitigation and adaptation are linked are the focus of this report.

Figure 2 expands upon the conceptual framework in Figure 1, and provides a global view of the complex ecological networks that can be disrupted by climate change, the human health implications of such disruptions, and the targets of mitigation and adaptation. Many

of these diseases[12] and disorders are not independently affected; any one disease is likely to have several drivers from the group of environmental consequences that result from climate change, and conversely, any particular environmental change could affect multiple disease categories. In addition, both positive and negative synergies will occur among various components of the system.

Climate change directly affects five components of the environment: water, air, weather, oceans, and ecosystems.[13] Changes in rainfall and other precipitation, changing temperatures, and melting of summer ice caps are already occurring and will create changes in the availability and quality of water across much of the planet over the next 30 years.[14] In the United States, water security, or the reliable availability of water for drinking, agriculture, manufacturing, and myriad other uses, is becoming a pressing issue. This is particularly true in the Western half of the country, where water shortages are exacerbated by reduced mountain snowpack due to warming, and in the South, where severe droughts have become a more frequent occurrence in recent years. Water quality is also affected in many regions, particularly coastal areas, due to extreme weather events

12 For simplicity, we will use disease to include the broad spectrum of human diseases, syndromes, ailments and conditions being described here.
13 Intergovernmental Panel on Climate Change. Working Group II. 2007. Cambridge: Cambridge University Press. ix, 976 p. Karl, T, et al. 2009. New York: Cambridge University Press.
14 Intergovernmental Panel on Climate Change. Working Group II. 2007. Cambridge: Cambridge University Press. ix, 976 p.

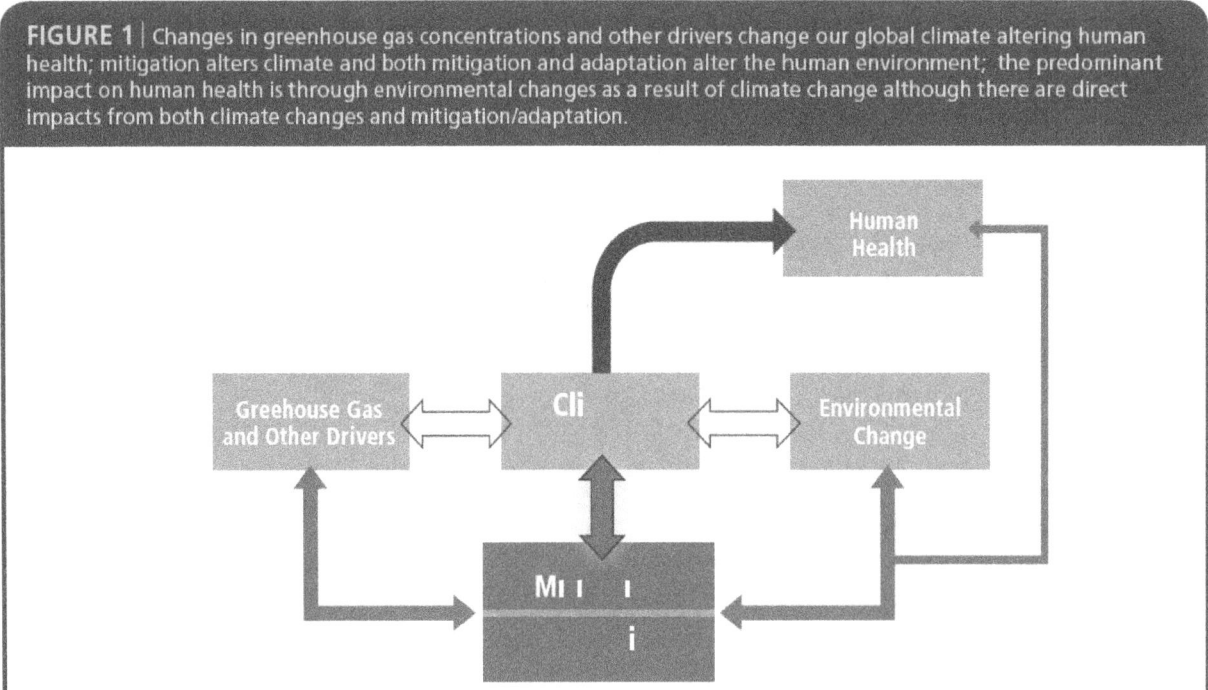

FIGURE 1 | Changes in greenhouse gas concentrations and other drivers change our global climate altering human health; mitigation alters climate and both mitigation and adaptation alter the human environment; the predominant impact on human health is through environmental changes as a result of climate change although there are direct impacts from both climate changes and mitigation/adaptation.

such as hurricanes and flooding. These same events, often associated with sea-level rise and increased storm surges, can heavily damage human communities and alter complex coastal ecosystems with consequences for both water and food quality and supply.

The complex atmospheric chemistry that governs air quality is modulated by heat, humidity, degree of ultraviolet (UV) radiation, and many other factors. Changes in any of these can directly reduce air quality, particularly in urban areas, by increasing air concentrations and human exposures to a variety of toxic air pollutants including chemicals, fungi, and aeroallergens. In many areas of the country, climate change and resulting weather events such as drought and wildfires will reduce general air quality and increase

human exposure to a variety of pollutants, with resulting increases in asthma, cardiovascular disease, and other respiratory ailments.

Some of the human health effects will arise from extreme weather events that are expected to become more common in a warmer climate. For instance, more intense hurricanes and increases in flooding and wildfires may exacerbate a wide range of health effects resulting from the release of toxic chemicals from landfills, contamination of drinking water with raw sewage as a result of damage to water infrastructure, increased concentrations of air pollutants that are especially harmful to susceptible populations such as children, the elderly, and those with asthma or cardiovascular disease, and myriad other hazards associated with these events. Extreme heat

FIGURE 2 | Climate change has direct impacts on five aspects of the human environment (red lines, purple circles) that in turn impact additional environmental factors. These environmental changes then alter twelve separate aspects of human health (tan boxes). Mitigation and adaptation alter the human environment in order to address climate change and, in this way, alter human health. Finally, susceptible populations exist for all climate-targeted health points, and the health systems play an integral role in addressing the health concerns driven by climate change.

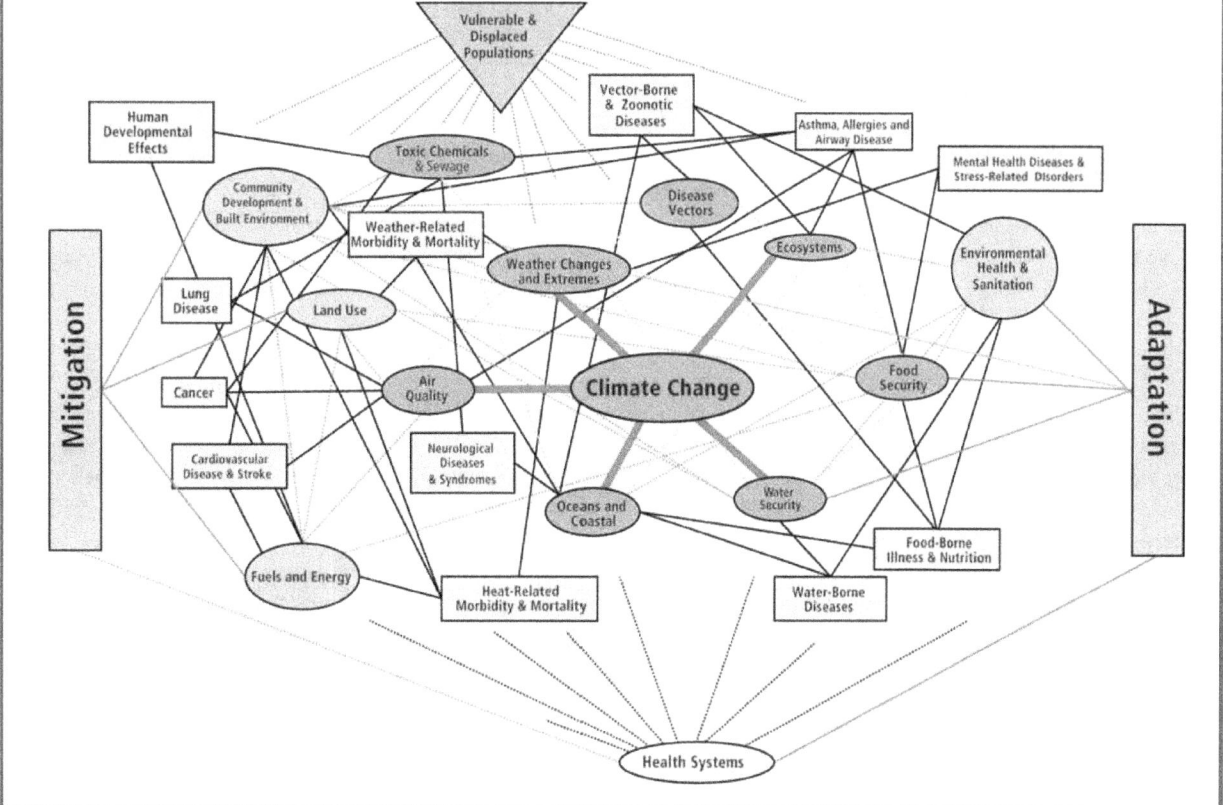

also directly increases the risk of injury, illness, and death, as well as indirectly by contributing to illnesses such as those associated with mental health and stress.[15]

Global climate change is visibly and profoundly affecting oceans, which in turn, affects human health. The warming of ocean waters contributes to increases in incidence and severity of toxic algal blooms, alterations in aquatic and estuarine food webs and seafood quality and availability, and effects on sentinel aquatic species[16]. High concentrations of carbon dioxide in the atmosphere increase the amount that is dissolved into the ocean, leading to acidification and disruption of ecosystems. As large portions of the world's populations, including those in the United States, live in coastal areas, and many depend on marine protein for daily subsistence, the consequences of perturbing delicate ocean and coastal systems will be far-reaching.

Climate changes including increased heat in certain arid and semi-arid parts of the United States can dramatically alter existing ecosystems, presenting new challenges to agricultural production and coastal ecosystems, with consequences for food quality and availability. Changes in plant habitat can result in reduced availability of grazing lands for livestock.[17] Climate changes also are directly associated with many pest habitats and disease vectors, and changes in temperature can extend or reorient habitats such that organisms are introduced to new geographic areas or life cycles are altered, requiring increases in pesticide use or use in new areas to achieve the same yields. Global warming is also causing shifts in the ranges of disease vectors that require specific environments to thrive (for example, Lyme disease),[18] and increasing the threat and incidence in humans of waterborne, vectorborne and zoonotic (those transferred from animals to humans) diseases.

No current mitigation strategy or technology can prevent the change in climate that has already occurred. At present, our ability to mitigate the magnitude of the climate changes that will occur over the next 100 years is limited by the current makeup of the atmosphere, as well as what we can prevent from entering and what we are able to remove from the atmosphere in the future. The major targets of climate change mitigation strategies include alternative fuels and energy conservation, changes in land use patterns, sustainable development of the built environment, and carbon capture and storage.[19] Switching from fossil fuels and other greenhouse

gas-emitting energy sources to cleaner alternatives and using carbon capture and storage technologies will slow the rate at which we release greenhouse gases into the environment. Energy conservation and modifications in energy use will also reduce releases. Land use changes such as restricting the destruction of forests and replanting more trees will serve to increase natural carbon storage.

Actions to preserve other ecosystem services, such as flood control by protecting wetlands or vector control by conserving biodiversity, can also reduce the severity of climate change-related problems.[20] Finally, changes in building codes, transportation infrastructure, housing density, coastal development, and other urban planning strategies can reduce energy usage and thereby mitigate some portion of climate change. Through these changes in human activities and practices, we should be able to limit the magnitude of the changes to the planet's climate, and thus, reduce the negative impacts to human health. Though it is possible that some mitigation strategies may exacerbate known human health stressors or introduce unanticipated potential for human harm, many strategies will provide co-benefits, simultaneously reducing the negative effects of climate change while also reducing illness and death. For example, reducing harmful air pollutants generally decreases global warming but is also just more healthful to people.[21]

Recognizing that there are a broad set of issues related to both potential benefits and possible adverse effects on human health resulting from mitigation and adaptation strategies, the IWGCCH did not attempt to outline research needs for mitigation and adaption in a comprehensive manner in this report, nor provide a comprehensive overview of mitigation and adaptation approaches. These issues and their associated research needs will have to be evaluated in the context of the individual options and strategies. Instead, this report focuses on some of the broader mitigation and adaptation options that are currently under development that have the potential to provide great benefits to human health and proposes research needs that could inform decisions relating to them, and examples of mitigation and adaptation needs related to certain health consequences are included within each chapter.

Adapting to or coping with climate change will become necessary in the United States and around the world. Most adaptation strategies seek to change the human environment and decrease the potential for illness and death by helping to prevent some of the worst consequences of climate change. The primary environmental factors targeted for adaptation are water security and food security.

15   Noyes, PD, et al., Environment International, 2009. 35(6): p. 971-986.
16   United States. Congress. Senate. Committee on Commerce Science and Transportation. 2003. Washington: U.S. G.P.O. II. 8 p.
17   Ericksen, PJ, et al., Environmental Science and Policy, 2009. 12(4): p. 373-377.
18   Estrada-Peña, A, Environ Health Perspect, 2002. 110(7): p. 635-40.
19   Haines, A, et al., Lancet, 2006. 367(9528): p. 2101-2109.

20   Corvalán, C, et al. 2005, [Geneva, Switzerland]: World Health Organization. 53 p.
21   Smith, KR, et al., Lancet, 2009.

Given the likely changes that will occur in precipitation patterns, temperature, and extreme weather events, adapting the ways in which we store, treat, and use water will be key to avoiding changes in water security. Similarly, food sources—whether they be crops, livestock, marine, or freshwater—will be under greater stress in various parts of the United States, and as a nation we need to develop adaptation strategies to ensure our food security. Clean water and access to sufficient safe food are fundamental needs for human health, so successful adaptation methods that maintain and improve the availability of clean water and healthy food will be critical to avoiding some of the major health impacts of climate change. There is also a need for adaptation strategies focused on community development and the built environment, transportation, and public health infrastructure.[22]

Through these environmental changes, increases—and in some rare cases—decreases in adverse human health consequences are likely to occur. We have organized these health consequences into 11 broad categories for discussion (listed below). In this report, we provide for each category a brief synopsis of what is known about the relationship between climate change; mitigation, and adaptation; effects on the risk, incidence, severity, or characteristics of the specific diseases or disorders; the major research needs and questions that must be addressed; and in some cases, an indication of the specific skills and capacities that will be needed to facilitate the research. Because factors including urgency, likelihood of occurrence, numbers of people affected, severity of effects, and economic issues associated with each category are broad, difficult to quantify, and largely beyond the mandate of our individual agencies, we have deliberately chosen not to attempt a prioritization of the research needs, but rather seek to provide a body of knowledge to inform federal agencies, and the government as a whole, as agencies and other groups set their own priorities and agendas in this area. The scope of this analysis is largely confined to examining effects on the U.S. population, which is the primary constituency of the federal agencies, recognizing that most, if not all, of these issues are of global concern and consequence as well, and in the hopes that resulting gains from this information can be applied to global collaborations in the future. Similarly, although we attempt to provide some discussion of the training, capacities, technology, and infrastructure needs that will be required to address these critical research questions, it is within the context and for the purpose of identifying and applying those resources present or anticipated within our specific federal agencies.

Finally, the health consequence categories, although treated as individual topics, are not discrete, but rather are connected through the complicated systems within our planet and our own bodies. We have tried to draw out these connections wherever possible and when they are of major significance. We also have identified a number of crosscutting issues that are critical to this discussion including susceptible, vulnerable, and displaced populations; public heath and health care infrastructure; capacities and skills needed; and communication and education to increase awareness of climate change health effects.

Categories of human health consequences of climate change:

1. Asthma, Respiratory Allergies, and Airway Diseases

2. Cancer

3. Cardiovascular Disease and Stroke

4. Foodborne Diseases and Nutrition

5. Heat-Related Morbidity and Mortality

6. Human Developmental Effects

7. Mental Health and Stress-Related Disorders

8. Neurological Diseases and Disorders

9. Vectorborne and Zoonotic Diseases

10. Waterborne Diseases

11. Weather-Related Morbidity and Mortality

---

22   Haines, A., et al., ibid 2006. 367(9528): p. 2101-2109.

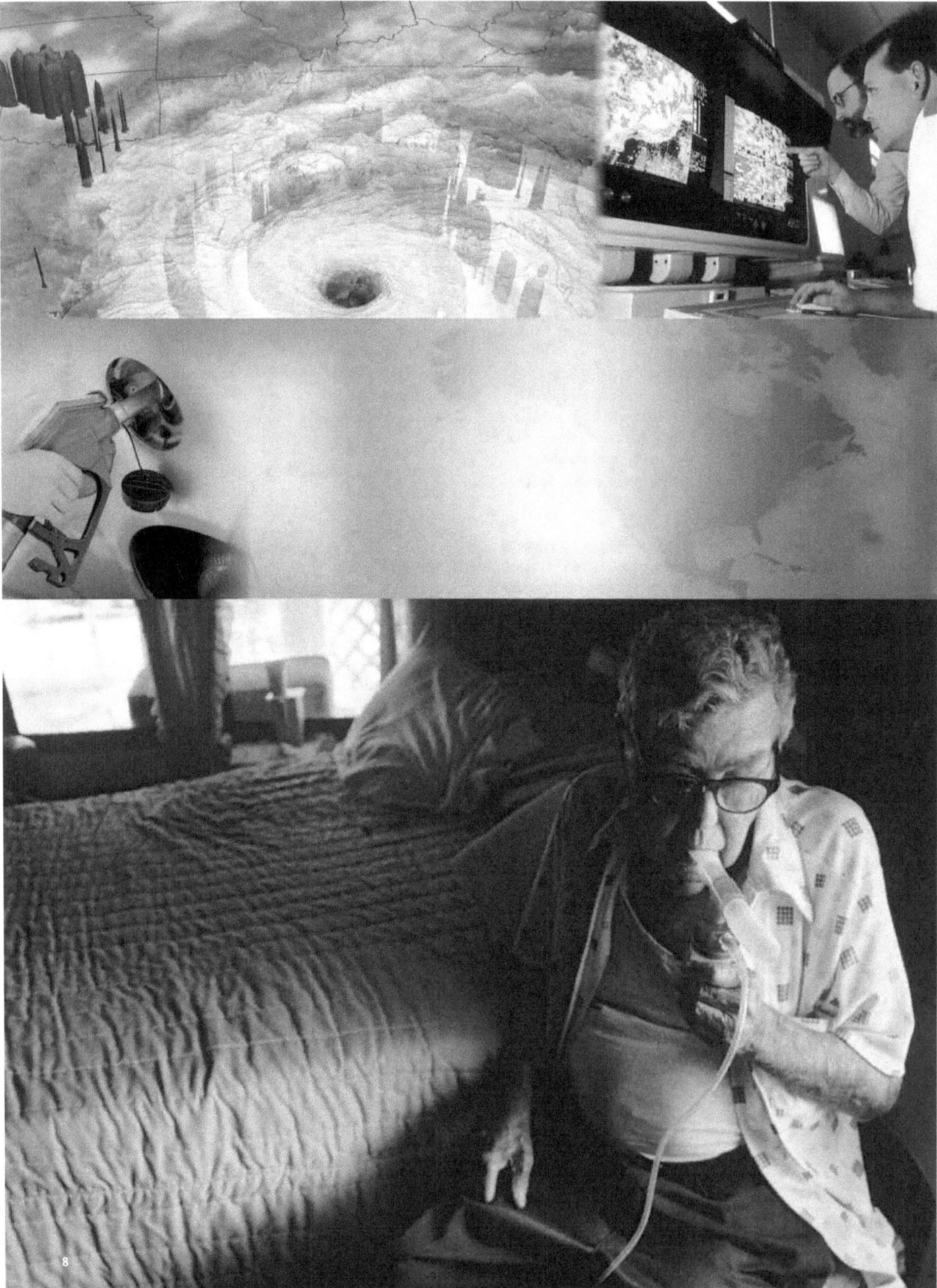

Crosscutting Issues for Climate Change and Health

In the process of identifying and characterizing research needs on the health implications of climate change for the 11 categories of consequences, it became evident that multiple crosscutting issues span all aspects of the research needs. In the sections below, we briefly summarize the major areas of overlap.

Susceptible, Vulnerable, and Displaced Populations. The World Health Organization defines "environment" as "all modifiable physical, chemical, and biological factors external to the human host, and all related behaviors that are critical to establishing and maintaining a healthy livable environment,"[23]. Within this definition, it is likely that the environment can affect most human diseases and illnesses. There are certain populations that are at increased risk from environmental factors that affect health, and such populations present unique concerns when considering the health risks from climate change. "Susceptibility" refers to intrinsic biological factors that can increase the health risk of an individual at a given exposure level. Examples of susceptibility factors that have been shown to increase individual health risks are certain genetic variants, life-stage such as childhood, and medical history such as a prior history of disease. "Vulnerability" refers to human populations at higher risk due to environmental or personal factors. For example, people living in mud brick houses in earthquake zones are much more vulnerable to injury from building collapse than those living in structures built with modern techniques and stronger materials. Populations living in poverty, substance abusers, and those with mental illness are at increased vulnerability to many of the environmental changes resulting from climate change. Another form of vulnerability is seen in displaced populations, who have been shown to be at higher risk of a number of diseases, including diarrheal and vectorborne diseases resulting from exposure to poor sanitation, as well as mental health illnesses due to increased acute and chronic stress.[24]

Populations with both susceptibility and vulnerability factors are referred to as "sensitive" populations. An example of a sensitive population would be certain members of the displaced population that evacuated New Orleans following Hurricane Katrina. Studies have shown that within this population, older people (susceptible)

who were of low income (vulnerable) were the slowest to recover from the disaster.[25] Virtually every human disease is likely to have both susceptible and vulnerable populations associated with it. One key aspect to mitigating the effects of climate change is a better understanding of diseases and the unique risks of various exposed or affected populations so that strategies may be developed that take such risks into account and are tailored to address them.

In the case of diseases linked to climate change, a number of populations are particularly at risk. Children, pregnant women, and the elderly are generally more susceptible, especially for heat- and weather-related illness and death, vectorborne and zoonotic diseases, and waterborne and foodborne illnesses.[26] Also, children and some minority groups are very susceptible to asthma and allergies that may be exacerbated by climate change. Genetic links and markers that help to identify and define susceptible populations exist for many climate-related diseases.

Poverty generally makes people more vulnerable to many of the health effects of climate change, largely due to inadequate access to health care. Poverty also increases the risk that a population displaced by extreme weather events or environmental degradation will not easily recover, and as a result, will suffer much higher disease risks. The same is true for people who abuse drugs, those who suffer mental illness, and others who for various reasons are socially isolated For such populations, the effects of climate change such as temperature and weather extremes, disruptions in access to public services including health care and food assistance programs, and increased stress are all magnified by their preexisting conditions or situations. Outdoor workers and people living in coastal and riverine zones also are likely to experience increased vulnerability to climate-induced environmental changes resulting from flooding and extreme weather events.

Data to support a broad understanding of which populations will be most susceptible and vulnerable to diseases affected by climate change are generally lacking at this time; however, data are

23   Prüss-Üstün, A. et al. 2006, Geneva, Switzerland: World Health Organization. 104 p.
24   Myers, N, Philos Trans R Soc Lond B Biol Sci. 2002. 357(1420): p. 609-13.
25   Eisenman, D.P. et al. Am J Public Health. 2007. 97 Suppl 1: p. S109-15.
26   Balbus, J.M, et al. Journal of occupational and environmental medicine / American College of Occupational and Environmental Medicine. 2009. 51(1): p. 33-37.

available that identify vulnerable populations for some diseases with environmental causes or triggers that are likely to be altered by climate change. For example, reducing vehicle emissions may mean that populations living near freeways, who are at higher risk of cardiovascular disease, asthma, and spontaneous abortion, may see a reduction in incidence of these effects.[27] Expanding research on these diseases to incorporate effects of climate change will help to identify vulnerable populations, and also to develop the strategies needed to adapt to climate changes and avoid excess health risks. These research efforts, if they are to be effective, must involve a broad spectrum of research scientists from epidemiologists and physicians to environmental engineers and community planners. Such efforts also will require a broad-based, multi-agency federal program that builds on the strengths of each agency to develop an overall comprehensive research agenda.

Public Health and Health Care Infrastructure. The term "public health" describes the science of preventing disease, prolonging life, and promoting health and its application to society, communities, and groups. In contrast, "health care" primarily focuses on the treatment of illness and the protection of mental and physical well being in individuals through services provided by physicians and other health care professionals. Together, these two areas are tasked with the protection of the health of the people of the United States.

Public health agencies exist across the United States in most large cities, as well as at the county, state, and federal levels. Schools of public health and other training and research institutions add to the total public health infrastructure investment of the United States, which is very large and quite complex. The public health system will play a critical role in the prevention of human disease from climate change. As such, public health agencies should be deeply involved in researching, developing, and implementing adaptation strategies to climate change. There is a critical need for research to understand how climate change will alter our public health needs in the United States, and to design optimal strategies to meet those needs.[28]

The health care delivery infrastructure in the United States is even more diverse and complicated than the public health infrastructure (though there are multiple overlaps between the two systems). From family doctors in small towns to complex university research

hospitals in large cities, health care professionals are the primary source of medical treatment, prenatal and pediatric care, and individual health protection and promotion for people in the United States. But this infrastructure is also vulnerable to climate change in a number of very important ways. Disasters can severely hinder the delivery of health care, with long-term impacts.[29] Changes in the numbers of patients and the spectrum of diseases with which they present could occur in some regions as the climate changes. The types of advice offered to patients with chronic conditions and the infrastructure to support them may need to be adapted to protect against climate-induced changes that may make these individuals more vulnerable. Currently there is limited research to guide these types of decisions.

The public health community is in the early stages of developing modeling skills and capacity in relation to climate change, particularly for combining climate models with ecological and other health outcome models for use in projecting disease dynamics under various climate scenarios. In order to understand these dynamics, a sustained surveillance infrastructure that integrates human and ecological health (terrestrial, marine, aquatic) is critical. While the public health community has developed considerable expertise in behavioral science and health education, this expertise has yet to be applied to the most trenchant issues related to climate change.

Sea-level rise, coastal erosion, and population displacement will create challenges for public health infrastructure that has been constructed over a period of hundreds of years. Disruption of coastal routes and harbors by sea-level rise will present additional challenges to health care delivery and food distribution. It is doubtful that transportation infrastructure will be able to adapt quickly enough to large population shifts that may be made in response to changes in rainfall patterns. Displaced populations will need sewer and water resources in new locations. The sewer and water resources in coastal locations may be threatened directly by sea-level rise.

Capacities and Skills Needed. Many of the existing skills used in public health and health care are well established and applicable to dealing with the health effects of climate change, but new skills will also be needed. Skills used in certain types of disease surveillance are well established. Less well established are the skills and methods needed to integrate current and future surveillance activities

27   Clougherty, JE, et al., Environ Health Perspect, 2009. 117(9): p. 1351-8; Green, RS, et al., Environ Health Perspect, 2009. 117(12): p. 1939-44.

28   Bedsworth, L, Environmental Health Perspectives, 2009. 117(4): p. 617-623.

29   Rudowitz, R, et al., Health Aff (Millwood), 2006. 25(5): p. w393-406.

and retrospective datasets with weather and climate information. Understanding of how to conceptualize and conduct epidemiological analysis using weather and climate as exposures is also preliminary. Methods and skill in combining spatial epidemiology with ecological approaches are also lacking. There is a strong need for the ability to translate vulnerability mapping and health impact assessments (HIAs) into behavioral changes and effective public health actions.

A greater emphasis must be placed on developing and maintaining interdisciplinary and inter-institutional collaborations, as well as on ensuring that established resources and expertise of all of the relevant disciplines, including climatology, modeling, environmental science, risk assessment, public health, and communications and education, are applied to these pressing problems. Many additional disciplines including ecology, social science, economics, geography, behavioral psychology, and others will need to play a vital role in climate and health decision making.

Communication and Education. Other areas where public health professionals may contribute robustly to efforts to address the impacts of climate change are in communication and education. Public health educators have a strong history of promoting health and wellness through educating individuals and communities about healthy behaviors and disease prevention or management. The same skills are critical to helping raise awareness of the potential impacts of climate change, and translating the scientific research and other technical data into credible and accessible information for the public to use in making informed decisions that will protect their health and the environment.

Recent studies show that the majority of those living in the United States now believe that climate change is a real and serious threat that is caused by human activity. However, research is still needed to determine how to effectively educate and organize the public to respond.[30] This is complicated by recent research showing that various audiences within the American public respond to the issue of climate change each in their own distinct way.[31] Research is needed that will aid climate change communicators and educators in adapting their messages and approaches to most appropriately and effectively reach and be assimilated by each individual audience.

In addition to the general public, other audiences—each with their own culture and means of acquiring information—also require effective communication on issues of climate change. Stakeholders such as natural resource managers, policy makers, infrastructure planners, health care providers, and others also need access to credible and timely climate change information to inform their decision-making.

Protecting human health is an issue that crosses institutional, scientific, and political boundaries. In the United States, no single institution at the local, regional, or federal level can fully protect public health without cooperation from other institutions. In addition, no single scientific field is capable of accomplishing all aspects of the research needed to understand the human health consequences of global climate change; such an endeavor will require a broad-based, trans-disciplinary research portfolio. And in our global society, the highly integrated activities of individuals around the world mean that no one country can be solely responsible for addressing the health impacts of global climate change. Through the process of developing this white paper, it rapidly became clear that identifying research needs; mobilizing and creating the expertise, resources, tools, and technologies to address them; and translating these efforts into solutions that will enable human adaptation to our changing environment while protecting public health will require collaborations on an unprecedented scale. Such collaborations should build on the strengths and capacities of individual organizations in ways that maximize the efforts of the group toward these shared goals.

30 Leiserowitz, A, et al., Climate change in the American mind: Americans' climate change beliefs, attitudes, policy preferences, and actions. 2009, Yale Project on Climate Change, Scool of Forestry and Environmental Sciences: New Haven, Connecticut. p. 56.

31 Maibach, E, et al., Global warming's six Americas 2009: An audience segmentation analysis. 2009, George Mason University Center for Climate Change Communication: Washington, DC. p. 140.

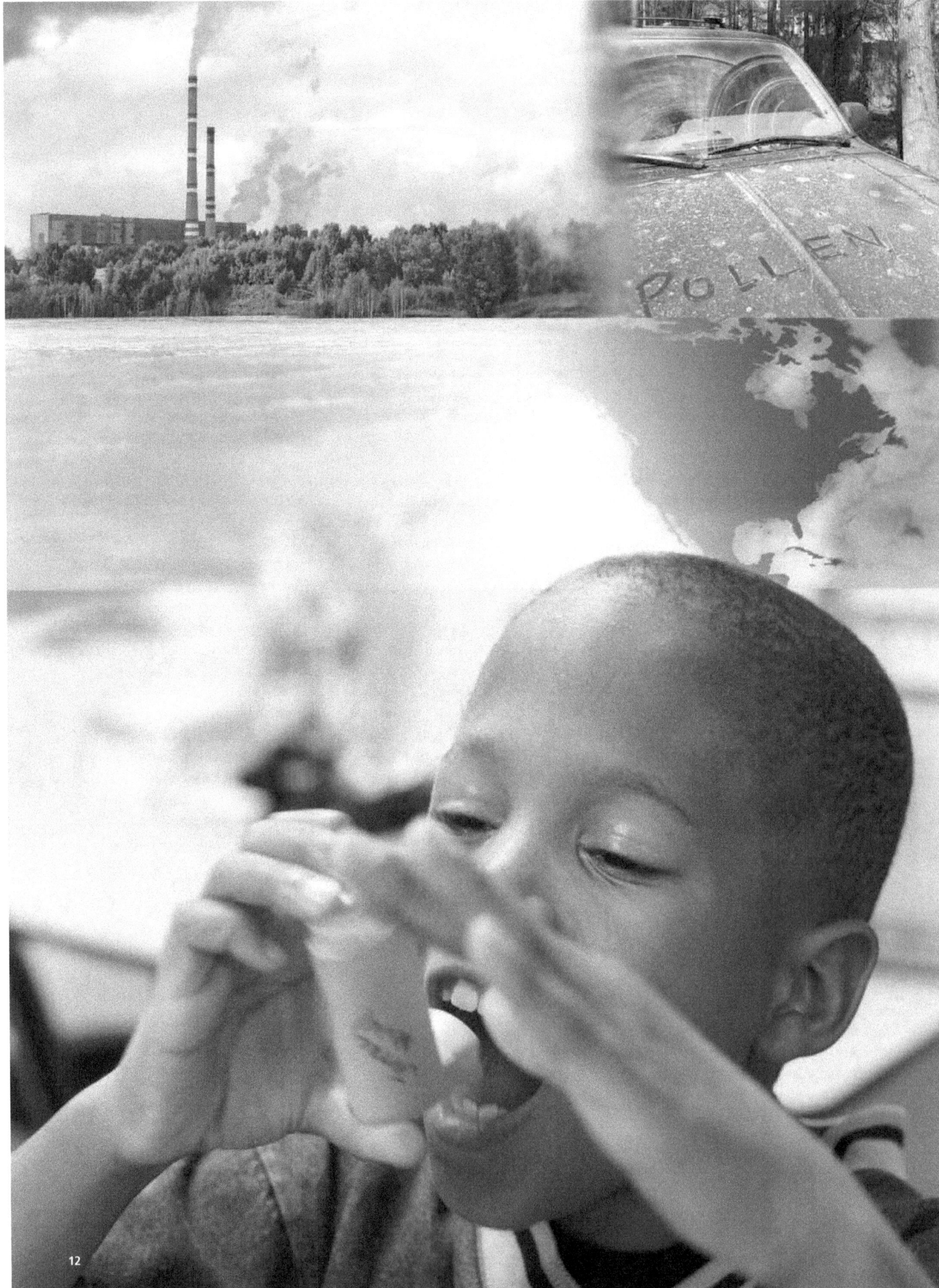

Asthma, Respiratory Allergies, and Airway Diseases

Allergic diseases, including asthma, hay fever, rhinitis, and atopic dermatitis, impact approximately 50 million individuals within the United States and are associated with significant health care costs and lost productivity.[32] In the early 1990s, the United States attributed health care costs of $11 billion to all respiratory disease with an estimated loss of 3 million workdays and 10 million schooldays.[33] Asthma is the second leading cause of chronic illness among children and is rapidly rising among children less than five years of age; however, the prevalence of asthma is highest among adults.[34] Incidence rates of asthma and other respiratory allergic diseases are often difficult to obtain; however rates of prevalence and disease exacerbation show a disproportionate trend along certain socioeconomic lines. Hospitalization rates, emergency department use, disability and death are often highest among children, African American and Hispanic populations, persons living in the inner city, and the poor.[35]

In recent decades, the world has seen a sharp rise in prevalence as well as severity of such respiratory diseases. The incidence of respiratory diseases grew markedly in the United States over the last several decades but has begun to plateau in recent years. Some experts speculate that the global rise in asthma was indirectly related to climate change.[36] Many respiratory allergic diseases are seasonal with climate sensitive components; climate change may increase the incidence and exacerbation of such allergic diseases. While some risk for respiratory disease can be clearly linked to climate change, for many others the risk attributable to climate change is unclear. Given the prevalence of these diseases and the significant disease burden imposed by asthma and respiratory allergic disease, further research into the impacts of climate change on these diseases should be a high priority.

Management of asthma and other respiratory allergic diseases relies on several factors including strict control of exacerbation triggers of the diseases. Although not all asthmatic episodes are triggered by environmental factors, a significant number are, including factors such as ambient air pollutants, allergens, stress, and a host of other environmental variables. As a result, changes to environment may adversely impact the severity of climate-sensitive diseases.

In addition to impacts on asthma and other allergic diseases, climate change has the potential to impact airway diseases by increasing ground level ozone and possibly fine particle concentrations. Breathing ozone can trigger a variety of reactions including chest pain, coughing, throat irritation, and congestion; and can worsen bronchitis, emphysema, and asthma. Exposure to ground-level ozone can also reduce lung function and inflame the linings of the lungs; repeated exposure may permanently scar lung tissue.[37] Fine particles (fewer than 2.5 micrometers in diameter, or $PM_{2.5}$) contain microscopic solids or liquid droplets that are so small that they can get deep into the lungs where they cause serious health problems. Numerous scientific studies have linked exposure to fine particle pollution to a variety of health problems including increased respiratory symptoms (irritation of the airways, coughing, difficulty breathing), decreased lung function, aggravated asthma, development of chronic bronchitis, irregular heartbeat, nonfatal heart attacks, and premature death in people with heart or lung disease.[38]

Impacts on Risk

Climate change will affect air quality through several pathways including production and allergenicity of aeroallergens such as pollen and mold spores and increases in regional ambient concentrations of ozone, fine particles, and dust. Some of these pollutants can directly cause respiratory disease or exacerbate respiratory disease in susceptible individuals.

Earlier flower blooming resulting from temperature increases and increased carbon dioxide (CO_2) concentrations affects timing of distribution of aeroallergens such as pollen through plant photosynthesis and metabolism.[39] There is also a possibility that certain aeroallergens may become more allergenic as temperatures and CO_2 concentrations increase.[40] Precipitation-affected aeroallergens such as mold spores also are of concern, as 5% of individuals are predicted to have some respiratory allergic airway symptoms from molds over their lifetime.[41]

32   Bytomski, JR, et al., Curr Sports Med Rep, 2003. 2(6): p. 320-4.
33   Smith, DH, et al., Am J Respir Crit Care Med, 1997. 156(3 Pt 1): p. 787-93; Weiss, KB, et al., N Engl J Med, 1992. 326(13): p. 862-6.
34   Benson, V, et al., Vital Health Stat 10, 1998(190): p. 1-428.
35   Mannino, DM, et al., MMWR CDC Surveill Summ, 1998. 47(1): p. 1-27A.
36   D'Amato, G, et al., Clinical and Experimental Allergy, 2008. 38(8): p. 1264-1274.

37   Uysal, N, et al., Curr Opin Pulm Med, 2003. 9(2): p. 144-50.
38   Kreyling, WG, et al., J Aerosol Med, 2006. 19(1): p. 74-83.
39   Stitt, M, Plant Cell and Environment, 1991. 14(8): p. 741-762.
40   Cassassa, G, et al. 2007, Cambridge: Cambridge University Press; Rogers, CA, et al., Environmental Health Perspectives, 2006. 114(6): p. 865-869; Shea, KM, et al., Journal of Allergy and Clinical Immunology, 2008. 122(3): p. 443-453; Vose, RS, et al., Nature, 2004. 427(6971): p. 213-214; Wan, SQ, et al., American Journal of Botany, 2002. 89(11): p. 1843-1846; Ziska, LH, et al., Global Change Biology, 2005. 11(10): p. 1798-1807.
41   Hardin, BD, et al., J Occup Environ Med, 2003. 45(5): p. 470-8.

In the presence of certain air emissions, the rate of ozone formation increases with higher temperatures and increased sunlight, and can also be affected by changes in storm tracks, humidity, and stability of the boundary layer (lowest part of the atmosphere).[42] Humidity and temperature also partly determine the formation of $PM_{2.5}$. Research studies associate fine particles with negative cardiovascular outcomes such as heart attacks, formation of deep vein blood clots, and increased mortality from several other causes.[43] These adverse health impacts intensify as temperatures rise.[44] Studies also link elevated exposure to ground-level ozone, $PM_{2.5}$, coarse thoracic PM, and aeroallergens to decreased lung function, aggravation of asthma, rhinitis, exacerbations of chronic obstructive pulmonary disease, hospitalizations for respiratory and cardiovascular diseases, and premature mortality.

Air pollution overcomes the mucosal barrier in lungs by inducing airway inflammation, which results in allergen-induced respiratory responses.[45] In addition, air pollutants such as $PM_{2.5}$ and ozone may alter the allergenicity of aeroallergens like pollen, thereby promoting further airway sensitization.[46] The triggers for such adverse respiratory responses vary and include climatic factors (meteorological events, rainfall patterns, and temperature anomalies), high levels of vehicle emissions, land-use patterns, variables in the built environment, geography, and distance from roadways.[47] Physiology also plays a significant role, as individuals with existing respiratory conditions are most vulnerable to disease exacerbations triggered by the environment.[48] The populations most vulnerable to the increased disease risks include children, pregnant women, persons of low socioeconomic status, persons situated near high traffic zones within urban centers, and those with preexisting respiratory and cardiovascular diseases.

Other airborne exposures are also likely to worsen with climate variability and change. Changes in the hydrologic cycle with increasingly variable precipitation and more frequent drought may also lead to a global increase of airborne dust, which, when coupled with anticipated stagnant air masses and increasingly strong inversion layers, will trap ozone and other airborne pollutants near the ground causing exacerbations of respiratory disease. Coarse thoracic PM (between 2.5 and 10 micrometers in diameter) is associated with increased risk of emergency department visits and hospitalizations for cardiovascular outcomes, especially among adults over 65 years of age.[49] Increased incidence of wildfires in some areas can also contribute to PM concentrations. In certain areas airborne dust serves as a carrier of specific diseases, such as coccidioidomycosis, or "valley fever," in the desert Southwest, the incidence of which has increased in recent years.[50] Prolonged drought will lead to more dust and particulate pollution while increased rainfall will cleanse the air but may create more mold and microbial pollution. In addition, drought, declining water quality, and increased temperatures contribute to the growth of harmful algal blooms that produce toxins that can be aerosolized and exacerbate asthma and respiratory diseases.[51]

Despite strong evidence of associations between a wide range of environmental variables impacted by climate and respiratory disease, the direct impacts of climate change on asthma, respiratory allergies, and airway diseases need further study to evaluate the fraction of respiratory disease risk that can be attributed to climate change and potentially mitigated or avoided.

Mitigation and Adaptation

Mitigation and adaptation strategies have the potential to both positively and negativel affect human health. Reduction of vehicle miles traveled will reduce ozone precursors, thereby reducing the ozone associated with myriad respiratory health effects. Alternative transportation options such as walking and bicycling will reduce toxic emissions while providing positive benefits for health such as increasing cardiovascular fitness and contributing to weight loss (although such activities also have the potential to increase exposure to harmful outdoor air pollutants, particularly in urban areas, simply by virtue of increased time spent outdoors)[52]. Mitigation of short-lived contaminant species that are both air pollutants and greenhouse gases is gaining momentum.[53] For example, controlling ozone or black carbon could bring short-term climate benefits and alleviate a fraction of the current health burden from these pollutants. Urban tree cover has been shown to reduce ambient concentrations of ozone, PM, and other pollutants.[54] Significant co-benefits of urban vegetation include shade, which reduces the heat-island effect and decreases energy required to cool buildings, and a concomitant reduction in greenhouse gas emissions.[55]

42 Houghton, JT, et al. 2001. Cambridge ; New York: Cambridge University Press. x, 881 p.

43 Bytomski, JR, et al., Curr Sports Med Rep, 2003. 2(6): p. 320-4, Vose, RS, et al., Nature, 2004. 427(6971): p. 213-214, Baccarelli, A, et al., Archives of Internal Medicine, 2008. 168(9): p. 920-927, Confalonieri, U, et al. in Climate Change 2007: Impacts, Adaptation and Vulnerability. Contribution of Working Group II to the Fourth Assessment Report of the Intergovernmental Panel on Climate Change, M Parry, et al., Editors. 2007, Cambridge University Press: Cambridge. p. 391-431, O'Neill, S, et al., Occupational and Environmental Medicine, 2007. 64(6): p. 373-379, Peters, A, et al., Circulation, 2001. 103(23): p. 2810-2815, Samoli, E, et al., Environmental Health Perspectives, 2008. 116(11): p. 1480-1486.

44 Qian, ZM, et al., Environmental Health Perspectives, 2008. 116(9): p. 1172-1178.

45 D'Amato, G, et al., Clinical and Experimental Allergy, 2008. 38(8): p. 1264-1274.

46 D'Amato, G, et al., Respiratory Medicine, 2001. 95(7): p. 606-611.

47 Shea, KM, et al., Journal of Allergy and Clinical Immunology, 2008. 122(3): p. 443-453.

48 D'Amato, G, et al., Clinical and Experimental Allergy, 2008. 38(8): p. 1264-1274.

49 Ballester, F, et al., Gac Sanit, 2006. 20 Suppl 1: p. 160-74, Le Tertre, A, et al., J Epidemiol Community Health, 2002. 56(10): p. 773-9, Zanobetti, A, et al., Environ Health Perspect, 2003. 111(9): p. 1188-93.

50 Komatsu, K, et al., Journal of the American Medical Association, 2003. 289(12): p. 1500-1502, Vugia, DJ, et al., Journal of the American Medical Association, 2009. 301(17): p. 1760-1762.

51 Abraham, WM, et al., Environmental Health Perspectives, 2005. 113(5): p. 632-637, Fleming, LE, et al., Chest, 2007. 131(1): p. 187-194.

52 Woodcock, J, et al., Lancet, 2009. 374(9705): p. 1930-43.

53 Smith, KR, et al., Ibid.

54 Bowker, G, et al., Atmospheric Environment, 2007. 41: p. 8128-8139, Nowak, D, et al., Urban Forestry and Urban Greening, 2006. 4: p. 115-123.

55 Bolund, P, et al., Ecological Economics, 1999. 29: p. 293-301, McPherson, E, et al., Urban Ecosystems, 1997. 1: p. 49-61.

Adaptive measures such as increased use of air conditioning may alleviate some of the health effects associated with exposure to chronic or acute heat, but also can potentially result in higher greenhouse gas emissions and further declines in air quality, depending on the method of power generation. Health-based research to inform the use of novel fuel mixtures and electric vehicles will be important. Some impacts have been well characterized through life-cycle analyses, while others, particularly those related to novel fuels and energy sources, have yet to be assessed. Careful analyses of mitigation and adaptation co-benefits and tradeoffs are necessary so that appropriate strategies are adopted.

Research Needs

Climate change will likely amplify existing environmental stimulation of asthma, respiratory allergies, and airway disease, resulting in more severe and frequent disease exacerbations and an increase in the overall burden of these conditions. Thus, continued research on climate change's effect on alterations in the composition of aeroallergens and air pollutant mixtures and their consequent effects on health is essential. Research needs include:

- developing and validating real-time remote sensing and other *in situ* monitoring techniques to evaluate air quality, aeroallergens, aerosolized pathogens, dust burdens, and other climate-sensitive exposures directly linked to asthma and airway diseases

- understanding and modeling the impact of climate change on air quality, aeroallergens, and aerosolized marine toxins, and the resulting effects on asthma and airway diseases including in vulnerable populations

- applying modeling originally developed to assess health effects of air pollution and other ecological niche modeling to climate-sensitive diseases

- establishing climate-sensitive exposure metrics, with appropriate temporal and spatial dimensions, that are most strongly associated with asthma, allergy, and airway diseases

- identifying and mapping populations and communities at increased risk of climate-related respiratory disease, which will also help to identify populations at risk for other climate-related health impacts as many environmentally mediated diseases share common risk factors

- using epidemiological investigations to study the relationship between climate variables; altered production, distribution, and reactivity of pollen and marine toxins; changes in air pollutants; and the prevalence, severity, and onset of asthma exacerbations

- studying the health effects of airborne and indoor dust on asthma exacerbation, including changes in dust composition resulting from climate change

- understanding the acute and long-term impacts of wildfires on asthma and other respiratory diseases

- examining chemicals used in energy efficient technologies to ensure that they do not contribute to lung sensitization, asthma, or other respiratory diseases

- examining the relative risks for respiratory disease based on chemicals with lower global warming potential than existing greenhouse gases

- developing early warning systems for state and local governments and public and environmental health officials to anticipate and mitigate climate-related health impacts

- improving methods of identifying risks and communicating with vulnerable populations to reduce climate change impacts on all respiratory diseases

- developing decision support tools including health impact assessments (HIAs) of the burden of respiratory diseases attributable to climate change for help in identifying and selecting climate change and air quality mitigation and adaptation policies that will promote health benefits

Research needs also call for improvements in various capacities and skills. Air pollution modeling is well established and the health impacts of several species of particles and aeroallergens are reasonably well understood. However, the complex introduction of aeroallergens under a changing climate will require the expansion of scientific expertise to include botany and ecology in addition to meteorology and the built environment. Research will require the use of geographic information systems (GIS) and remote sensing expertise in new ways, as well as the application of novel vulnerability mapping techniques, early warning systems, and other public health tools. Spatial epidemiological methods will bring new power to ecological studies of air quality and public health. Identification and collection of integrated and appropriately scaled social, ecological, and epidemiological data are needed for effective monitoring and modeling. For health communications, novel strategies are required to identify vulnerable populations and develop communication strategies that will effectively reduce risk.

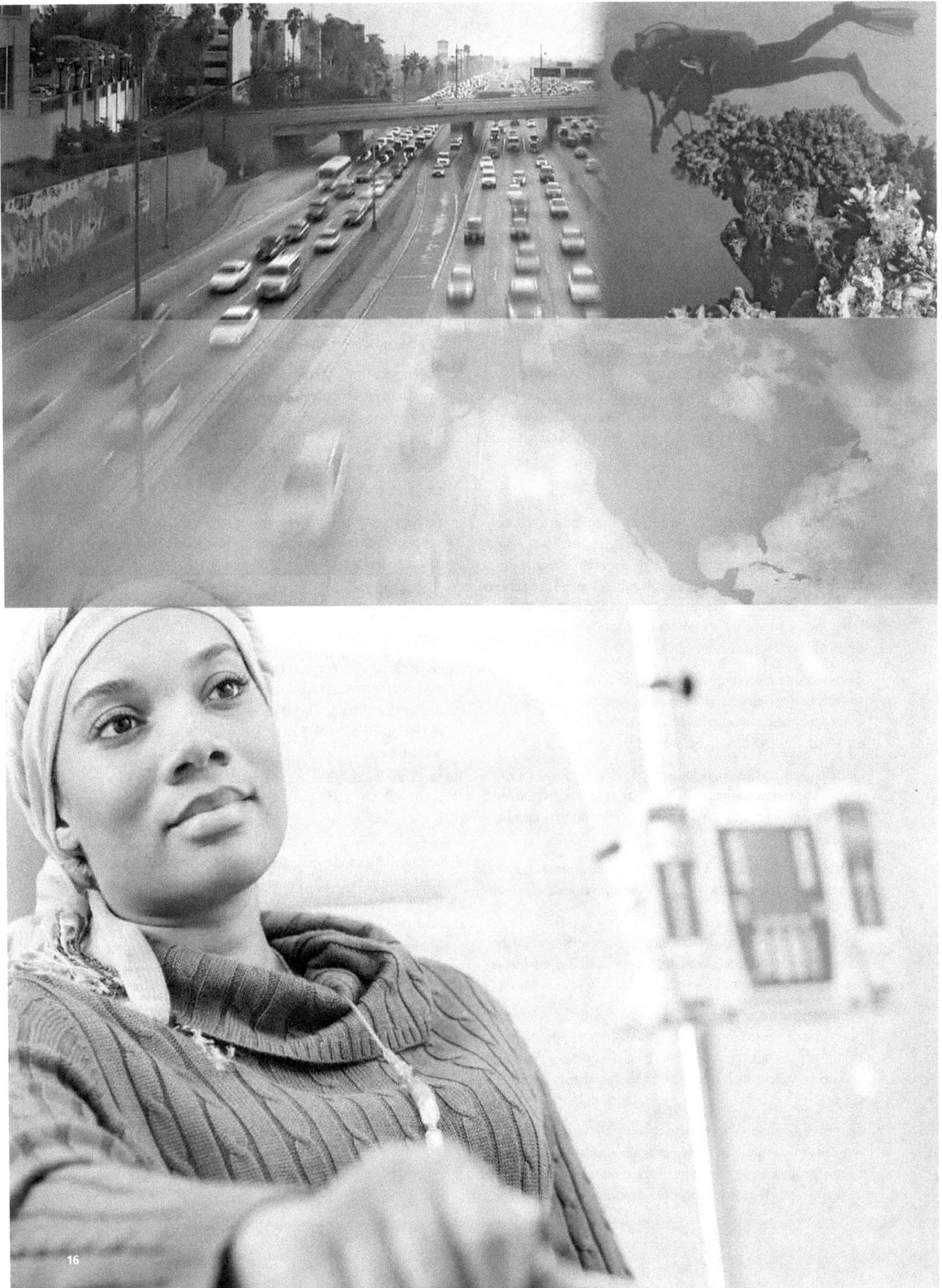

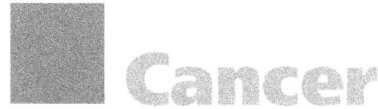

Cancer

Cancer refers to a group of diseases in which abnormal cells divide without control and are able to invade other tissues. There are more than 100 different types of cancer, and they are generally referred to by the organ or type of cell in which they arise (e.g. breast, prostate, colon). Cancer is the second leading cause of death in the United States after heart disease, killing more than half a million people every year.[56] Lung cancers, with about 220,000 new cases per year and about 160,000 deaths,[57] account for about 30% of overall deaths from cancer in the United States.[58] The main cause of lung cancer is smoking, especially cigarettes, but air pollution,[59] including indoor air pollution[60] and fine particulates,[61] also contributes to the burden of lung cancers.

There are potential impacts on cancer both directly from climate change and indirectly from climate change mitigation strategies. Climate change will result in higher ambient temperatures that may increase the transfer of volatile and semi-volatile compounds from water and wastewater into the atmosphere, and alter the distribution of contaminants to places more distant from the sources, changing subsequent human exposures.[62] Climate change is also expected to increase heavy precipitation and flooding events, which may increase the chance of toxic contamination leaks from storage facilities or runoff into water from land containing toxic pollutants. Very little is known about how such transfers will affect people's exposure to these chemicals—some of which are known carcinogens—and its ultimate impact on incidence of cancer.[63] More research is needed to determine the likelihood of this type of contamination, the geographical areas and populations most likely to be impacted, and the health outcomes that could result.

Although the exact mechanisms of cancer in humans and animals are not completely understood for all cancers, factors in cancer development include pathogens, environmental contaminants, age, and genetics. Given the challenges of understanding the causes of cancer, the links between climate change and cancer are a mixture of fact and supposition, and research is needed to fill in the gaps in what we know.

Impacts on Risks

One possible direct impact of climate change on cancer may be through increases in exposure to toxic chemicals that are known or suspected to cause cancer following heavy rainfall and by increased volatilization of chemicals under conditions of increased temperature. In the case of heavy rainfall or flooding, there may be an increase in leaching of toxic chemicals and heavy metals from storage sites and increased contamination of water with runoff containing persistent chemicals that are already in the environment. Marine animals, including mammals, also may suffer direct effects of cancer linked to sustained or chronic exposure to chemical contaminants in the marine environment, and thereby serve as indicators of similar risks to humans.[64] Climate impact studies on such model cancer populations may provide added dimensions to our understanding of the human impacts.

Another direct effect of climate change, depletion of stratospheric ozone, will result in increased ultraviolet (UV) radiation exposure. UV radiation exposure increases the risk of skin cancers and cataracts.[65] The incidence of typically nonlethal basal cell and squamous cell skin cancers is directly correlated to the amount of exposure to UV radiation. This effect is compounded by several other variables including temperature and exposure to other compounds that can amplify the carcinogenic potential of UV radiation.[66] Rising temperatures (such as occur at night versus day and in summer versus winter) are associated with increases in UV exposure. If increases in average or peak temperatures occur as a result of climate change, an increase in the incidence of non-melanoma skin cancers may occur.[67] Previous studies have shown that increased UV radiation exposure combined with certain polycyclic aromatic hydrocarbons (PAHs) can enhance

56   National Cancer Institute. What is cancer?. 2009 [cited 2009 July 21]; Available from: http://www.cancer.gov/cancertopics/what-is-cancer.
57   National Cancer Institute. Lung Cancer. 2009 [cited 2009 July 26]; Available from: http://www.cancer.gov/cancertopics/types/lung.
58   Centers for Disease Control and Prevention. Leading causes of death, 2006. 2009 [cited 2009 July 22]; Available from: http://www.cdc.gov/nchs/FASTATS/lcod.htm.
59   Beelen, R, et al., Epidemiology, 2008. 19(5): p. 702-10.
60   Ibid.
61   Krewski, D, et al., Res Rep Health Eff Inst, 2009(140): p. 5-114; discussion 115-36. Pope, CA, 3rd, et al., JAMA, 2002. 287(9): p. 1132-41.
62   Macdonald, RW, et al., Human and Ecological Risk Assessment, 2003. 9(3): p. 643-660.
63   Bates, B, et al., Climate change and water. 2008, Intergovernmental Panel on Climate Change: Geneva. p. 210.

64   McAloose, D, et al., Nat Rev Cancer, 2009. 9(7): p. 517-26.
65   Tucker, MA, Hematol Oncol Clin North Am, 2009. 23(3): p. 383-95, vii.
66   Burke, KE, et al., Toxicol Ind Health, 2009. 25(4-5): p. 219-24.
67   van der Leun, JC, et al., Photochem Photobiol Sci, 2008. 7(6): p. 730-3.

the phototoxicity of these compounds and damage DNA.[68] However, it is also possible that increased exposure to UV radiation could elevate levels of circulating Vitamin D, which has been associated with a decreased risk for certain cancers such as colorectal cancer.[69] Increased UV radiation also could impact the human immune system and alter the body's ability to remove the earliest mutant cells that begin the cancer process, although it is unclear whether these changes would be beneficial or detrimental.[70]

Mitigation and Adaptation

In addition to direct impacts of climate change on cancer, the impact of mitigation strategies on cancer should also be considered. For instance, co-benefits of decreased greenhouse gas emissions and decreased cancer incidence may be attainable with energy efficient power generation and reduced emissions through lower vehicle miles traveled. These benefits could be realized through decreases in toxic outputs of fossil fuel-based power generation and transportation, including sulfur oxide and particulate matter (PM), which have been implicated in lung cancer.[71]

Decreases in greenhouse gas emissions are generally associated with decreases in cancers that occur due exposure to such pollutants. Increased energy efficiency will lead to reductions in emissions of sulfur dioxide, nitrous oxides, and PM, which should lead to reductions in rates of premature death including from certain cancers.[72] In most cases, these emission reductions will also result in subsequent reductions in ambient concentrations of ozone and secondary $PM_{2.5}$, which have been implicated in a variety of health effects including lung cancer. Reductions in other hazardous air pollutants, such as heavy metals from power generation and industrial processes that are known or suspected to cause cancer or other serious health effects, may also occur.

Several technologies currently being pursued to decrease greenhouse gas emissions may also help to reduce cancer incidence. For example, reducing greenhouse gas emissions from the transportation sector may be accomplished by reducing vehicle miles traveled through a variety of approaches such as high-density development, preservation of green space, and widespread use of mass transit. However, the impacts of some mitigation technologies on cancer have not been fully explored.

For example, nanotechnology may be promising for mitigating climate change through its use in efficient hydrogen powered vehicles, enhanced and cheaper solar power technology, and the development of a new generation of batteries and supercapacitors, yet little is known about potential links to cancer and other health outcomes.

New technologies have been proposed to decrease our dependence on greenhouse gas-intensive power generation and fuel use. However, many of these have potential impacts on cancer that should be more fully investigated prior to being implemented. The widespread adoption of biofuels may have unintended consequences including possible increases or decreases in cancer due to a change in the level of existing pollutants or the creation and emissions of new air pollutants.[73] Also, barring changes in agricultural practices, there is potential for increased pesticide use for the growth of certain biofuels such as corn ethanol. Exposure to some legacy pesticides has been implicated for cancer in both adults and children,[74] leading to current efforts by the EPA to avoid this problem in new products.

Research is needed to understand if there are cancer implications from the use of electric vehicles, including the production and disposal of portable electric storage systems. Manufacturing of batteries for electric cars and photovoltaic (solar) power systems may have consequences including increased exposure to metals. The most common type of battery currently in use is the nickel-metal-hydride (NiMH) battery, with other types of batteries (lithium ion, lithium ion polymer, valve regulated lead acid, and nickel-cadmium) also under development for vehicle use. Increased use of NiMH batteries will necessarily require significant increases in nickel production and the impacts associated with nickel mining and refining. High-level nickel exposure is associated with increased cancer risk, respiratory disease, and birth defects; the same is true with certain other metals, especially cadmium and lead.

Increased production of solar cells also can lead to increased environmental risks.[75] For example, cadmium-tellurium (CdTe) compounds in photovoltaic systems and the potential for increased cadmium emissions from mining, refining, and the manufacture, utilization, and disposal of photovoltaic modules. Cadmium and cadmium compounds like CdTe are classified as known human carcinogens

68   Dong, S., et al., Chem Res Toxicol, 2000. 13(7): p. 585-93; Toyooka, T., et al., Environ Mol Mutagen, 2006. 47(1): p. 38-47.
69   Garland, CF., et al., Ann Epidemiol, 2009. 19(7): p. 468-83.
70   Skeiffers, A., et al., J Immunotoxicol, 2004. 1(1): p. 3-14.
71   Pope, CA. 3rd, et al., JAMA, 2002. 287(9): p. 1132-41.
72   Woodcock, J, et al., Lancet, 2009. 374(9705): p. 1930-43; Haines, A., et al., Lancet, 2009; Wilkinson, P, et al., Lancet, 2009. 374(9705): p. 1917-29.

73   Hill, J., et al., Proceedings of the National Academy of Sciences of the United States of America, 2009. 106(6): p. 2077-2082.
74   Flower, KB, et al., Environ Health Perspect, 2004. 112(5): p. 631-5; Kang, D, et al., Environ Res, 2008. 107(2): p. 271-6; Mahajan, R, et al., Environ Health Perspect, 2006. 114(12): p. 1838-42.
75   Fthenakis, V. in Practical handbook of photovoltaics : fundamentals and applications, T. Markvart, et al., Editors. 2003, Elsevier Advanced Technology: New York; Fthenakis, VM, et al., Environ Sci Technol, 2008. 42(6): p. 2168-74.

by the National Toxicology Program and the International Agency for Research on Cancer and as probable human carcinogens by the EPA.[76] Acute exposure to CdTe can result in respiratory irritation and toxicity. Some of the other hazardous materials present in solar manufacturing include arsenic compounds, carbon tetrachloride, hydrogen fluoride, hydrogen sulfide, lead, and selenium compounds,[77] many of which have been linked with multiple health effects, including cancer.

Production of hydrogen fuel cells will require significant increases in the total amount of platinum consumed worldwide, with a similar increase in mining and the environmental impacts associated with mining, processing, and transport. If hydrogen is used in a significant way as a transportation fuel, consideration must be given to the impacts of emissions from leaks during production, fueling, and operation. Increased hydrogen leaks could result in stratospheric ozone depletion by up to 20%,[78] which could lead to increased incidence of skin cancer.

For mitigation of climate change, nuclear power has been suggested as a possible alternative to coal-based power generation. Although the risks associated with direct exposure to radiation from nuclear power generation have been below accepted danger levels throughout the industry's history, the human health consequences over the full nuclear energy life cycle (production through waste disposal) may be of greater concern.[79]

Heatlth Impact Assessments (HIAs) are a useful emerging strategy for evaluating the health effects of novel policies and technologies at various scales, and have already been applied to several potential climate change mitigation strategies.[80] Given the widespread uncertainty regarding the potential health impacts, including cancer, of certain mitigation strategies, HIAs can be a valuable tool for evaluating possible health effects, especially when used in combination with other approaches to life-cycle assessment.

Research Needs

Many of the cancer risks resulting from the direct effects of climate change have been fairly well studied. The largest research gaps are in the materials and methods used for mitigation and adaptation, and

their potential to increase or decrease cancer risks. Research needs include:

- utilizing animal cancer surveillance and investigations as sentinel biomedical models to better understand the environmental factors, mechanisms, and pathways of mammalian cancer risk

- developing and sustaining facilities and expertise to rapidly assess and monitor the threat of previously unrecognized toxins, carcinogens, and other bioactive molecules produced in response to stress on marine environments

- understanding the impact of increased heavy precipitation and flooding events on the risk of toxic contamination of the environment from storage facilities or runoff from land containing toxic chemicals, including the geographical areas, ecosystems, and populations most likely to be impacted and the health outcomes that could result

- understanding how climate changes such as changes in temperature and precipitation affect exposure to toxic chemicals including volatile and semi-volatile compounds and known or suspected human carcinogens

- elucidating the effects of ambient temperature on UV radiation-induced skin cancers, including the amplification of non-melanoma skin cancers

- evaluating the potential cancer risks through the entire life cycle of biofuel production, including risks from novel air pollutants and changes in agricultural practices that may increase exposures to pesticides, herbicides, and other environmental contaminants

- understanding cancer risks from the life cycle emissions of carcinogens and untested compounds associated with alternative energy and transportation technologies, particularly electricity storage systems and photovoltaic systems

- clarifying the life cycle cancer risks of nuclear energy radiation, including through occupational and environmental exposures

- developing mechanisms to conserve and explore marine and terrestrial biodiversity in environments likely to yield cancer cures and treatments

- characterizing and quantifying changes in cancer rates from implementation of specific greenhouse gas mitigation strategies, especially for existing fossil fuel-based energy production and use

76 Rep Carcinog. 2005(11): p. 1-A32.
77 Fthenakis, V. in Practical handbook of photovoltaics : fundamentals and applications, T Markvart, et al., Editors. 2003, Elsevier Advanced Technology: New York.
78 Tromp, TK, et al., Science. 2003. 300(5626): p. 1740-2.
79 Massachusetts Institute of Technology. 2003, [Boston MA]: MIT. x, 170 p.
80 Patz, J, et al., Health impact assessment of global climate change: Expanding on comparative risk assessment approaches for policy making. in Annual Review of Public Health. 2008. p. 27-39.

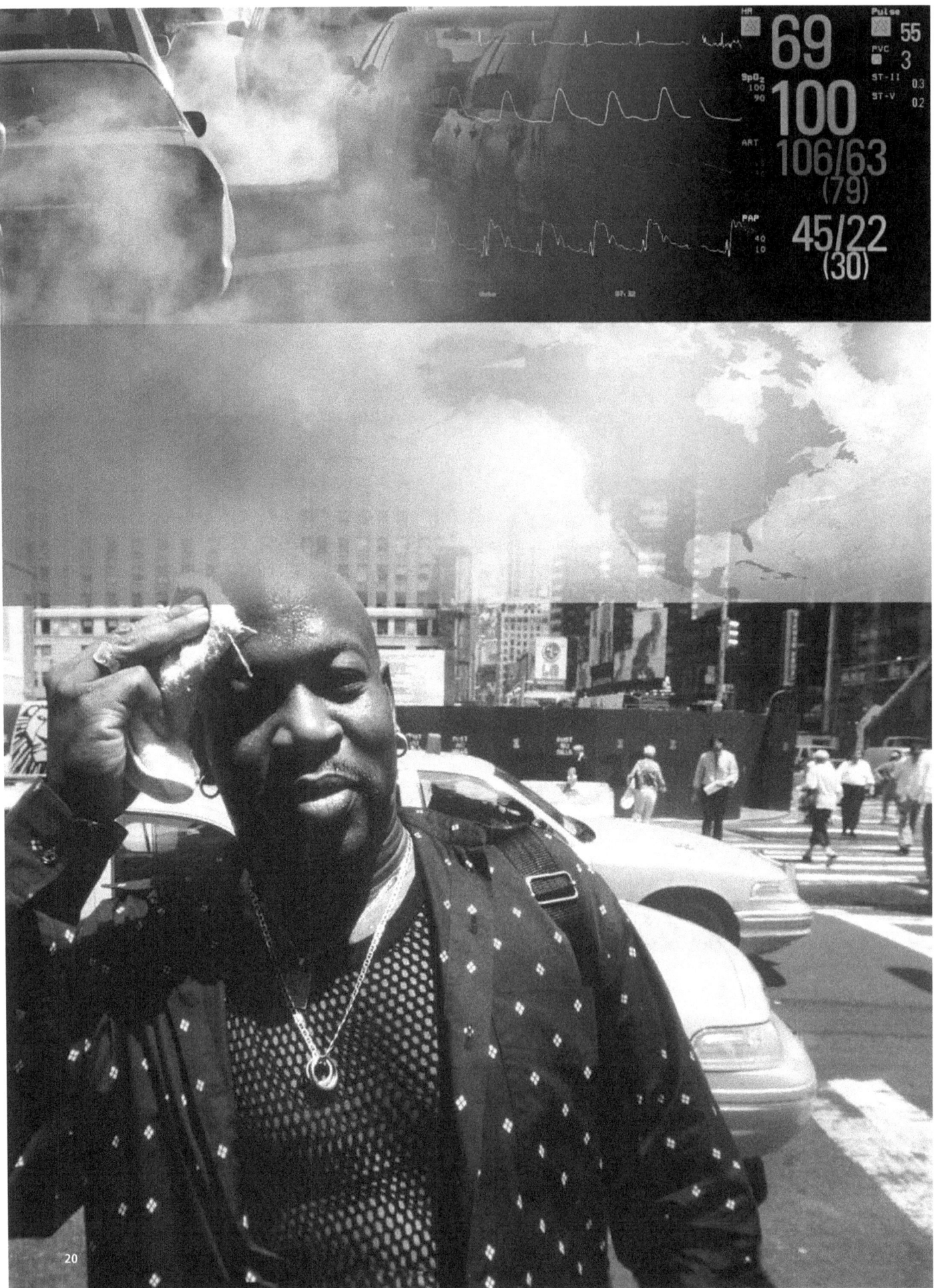

69
Pulse 55
3
100
106/63
(79)
45/22
(30)

20

Cardiovascular Disease and Stroke

Cardiovascular disease refers to a class of diseases that pertain to the heart or blood vessels. Cardiovascular disease is the leading cause of death in the United States, with 631,636 deaths in 2006, the last year for which statistics are available. Stroke is the third leading cause, with 131,119 deaths in 2006.[81] Approximately 80 million Americans have some form of cardiovascular disease including hypertension, coronary artery disease, heart attack, or stroke.[82] Other cardiovascular diseases such as cardiac dysrhythmias (abnormal electrical activity in the heart), deep venous thrombosis (blood clots), and pulmonary embolism (blood clots in the lung) increase the numbers further. The American Heart Association and the National Heart, Lung, and Blood Institute together estimate that cardiovascular disease will be responsible for $475.3 billion in direct and indirect health care expenditures in 2009.[83] Altogether, this diverse set of conditions is a major driver of health care expenditures and disability.

There is evidence of climate sensitivity for several cardiovascular diseases, with both extreme cold and extreme heat directly affecting the incidence of hospital admissions for chest pain, acute coronary syndrome, stroke, and variations in cardiac dysrhythmias, though the reported magnitude of the exposure-outcome associations is variable.[84] Weather conditions such as extreme heat serve as stressors in individuals with pre-existing cardiovascular disease, and can directly precipitate exacerbations.[85] There is also evidence that heat amplifies the adverse impacts of ozone and particulates on cardiovascular disease. These pollutants are likely to be affected by climate change mitigation activities, and thus, likely reduce rates of cardiovascular morbidity and mortality. While the fraction of disease risk attributable to weather and associated environmental exposures is not known, given the prevalence of cardiovascular disease and the preventable nature of the exposures, further research into associations between weather, climate variability, long-term climate change, and cardiovascular disease is an immediate need.

Impacts on Risk

Cardiovascular mortality associated with heat has been declining over time, presumably the result of increased air conditioning use; mortality associated with extreme cold has remained constant.[86] Cardiovascular hospital admissions increase with heat.[87,88] Dysrhythmias are primarily associated with extreme cold,[89] though associations with dysrhythmias and heat illness have been reported.[90] Stroke incidence increases with increasing temperature, as well.[91] For all direct associations between temperature and cardiovascular disease and stroke, elderly and isolated individuals are at greatest risk.

Indirect impacts of weather, weather variability, and climate changes on cardiovascular disease are many and varied. Associations between air quality, especially ozone and particulate burdens, and cardiovascular disease appear to be modified by weather and climate. Ozone, whose formation increases with temperature, increases cardiac effort and impairs pulmonary gas exchange.[92] Ozone concentrations modify the association between temperature and cardiovascular mortality,[93] and are also associated with acute myocardial infarction[94] (as discussed in the chapter on Asthma, Respiratory Allergies, and Airway Diseases). Particulate matter is associated with a variety of pathophysiological changes including systemic inflammation, deranged coagulation and thrombosis, blood vessel dysfunction and atherosclerotic disease, compromised heart function, deep venous thromboses,[95] and pulmonary embolism.[96] Increased burden of $PM_{2.5}$ is associated with increased hospital admissions and mortality from cardiovascular disease,[97] as well as ischemic heart disease.[98]

Other climate-related exposures are indirectly associated with incidence of cardiovascular disease and disease exacerbations.

81. Centers for Disease Control and Prevention. Leading causes of death, 2006. 2009 [cited 2009 July 22]; Available from: http://www.cdc.gov/nchs/FASTATS/lcod.htm.
82. American Heart Association. Cardiovascular disease statistics, 2006. 2009 [cited 2009 July 22]; Available from: http://www.americanheart.org/presenter.jhtml?identifier=4478.
83. American Heart Association. Cardiovascular disease cost, 2009. 2009 [cited 2009 July 22]; Available from: http://www.americanheart.org/presenter.jhtml?identifier=4475.
84. Bassil, KL, et al., Environmental Research. 2009. 109(5): p. 600-606; Kilbourne, EM, Am J Prev Med, 1999. 16(4): p. 359-60; McGeehin, MA, et al., Environ Health Perspect. 2001. 109 Suppl 2: p. 185-9, Pheer, WT, et al., Environ Health Perspect, 1999. 107(11): p. 911-6, Ye, F, et al., Environ Health Perspect, 2001. 109(4): p. 355-9.
85. Fouillet, A, et al., International Archives of Occupational and Environmental Health, 2006. 80(1): p. 16-24, Wainwright, S, et al., American Journal of Epidemiology, 1994. 139(11): p. 549-549.
86. Barnett, AG, Epidemiology, 2007. 18(3): p. 369-72.
87. Ebl, KL, et al., Int J Biometeorol, 2004. 49(1): p. 48-58, Morabito, M, et al., International Journal of Cardiology, 2005. 105(3): p. 288-293.
88. Schwartz, J, et al., Epidemiology, 2004. 15(6): p. 755-761.
89. Kysely, J, et al., BMC Public Health, 2009 Jan 15;9:19.
90. al-Harthi, SS, et al., Int J Cardiol, 1992. 37(2): p. 151-4.
91. Ebl, KL, et al., Int J Biometeorol, 2004. 49(1): p. 48-58.
92. Gong, H, et al., American Journal of Respiratory and Critical Care Medicine, 1998. 158(2): p. 538-546.
93. Ren, C, et al., Occupational and Environmental Medicine, 2008. 65(4): p. 255-260.
94. Ruldavets, JB, et al., Circulation, 2005. 111(5): p. 563-569.
95. Baccarelli, A, et al., Archives of Internal Medicine, 2008. 168(9): p. 920-927.
96. Brook, RD, Clinical Science, 2008. 115(6): p. 175-187.
97. Jerrett, M, et al., New England Journal of Medicine, 2009. 360(11): p. 1085-1095.
98. Pope, CA, et al., Journal of the Air & Waste Management Association, 2006. 56(6): p. 709-742.

Extreme weather events affect cardiovascular health through several pathways. Directly, the stress of the event and anxiety over event recurrence are associated with myocardial infarction,[99] sudden cardiac death,[100] and development of stress-related cardiomyopathy.[101] Indirectly, displacement related to disasters is frequently associated with interruptions of medical care for chronic medical conditions,[102] putting populations with chronic cardiovascular conditions at risk for disease exacerbations.

Climate is also implicated in another indirect risk for cardiovascular disease: the incidence of certain vectorborne and zoonotic diseases (VBZD) with cardiovascular manifestations. One estimate holds that approximately 10% of strokes in the developing world are related to exposure to certain VBZD,[103] many of which are climate sensitive. In particular, Chagas disease is an important cause of stroke worldwide (although not in the United States); 20 million people globally have chronic Chagas, which is an independent risk factor for stroke in Latin America[104] and a leading cause of heart failure in South America.[105] There is some evidence of climate sensitivity for Chagas disease,[106] though the topic is little studied. In the United States, Lyme disease is a prevalent vectorborne disease that has cardiovascular manifestations,[107] though the incidence of such manifestations is much lower than that associated with Chagas disease.

There is little published literature on the projected direct and indirect impacts of climate change on cardiovascular disease incidence. Many of the studies coupling down-scaled climate projections with health outcomes have examined a particular exposure, such as heat or ozone, and projected mortality based on known associations, but do not make specific projections as to the incidence of cardiovascular morbidity and mortality. Insofar as climate change will bring increased ambient temperatures, increasingly variable weather, and increased extreme events, we can infer that climate change will likely have an overall adverse impact on the incidence of cardiovascular disease. Similarly, the impact of climate change on the incidence of cardiovascular complications from extreme weather events and certain VBZD is also likely to increase. However, the magnitude of these effects and the degree to which they can be lessened with adaptation efforts is unclear and warrants much further study.

Mitigation and Adaptation

The likely impacts of climate change mitigation activities on risk of cardiovascular disease and stroke depend primarily on emissions-associated energy production activities, particularly in the transportation sector. Some mitigation activities related to energy production, such as the increased use of wind, wave, solar, and nuclear sources of power generation, are likely to reduce cardiovascular disease risks by reducing particulate and other air pollution emissions.

Mitigation activities such as increasing the density of urban development, enhancing public transportation options, and encouraging alternatives to single occupancy vehicle use are likely to benefit cardiovascular fitness, reducing the overall burden of cardiovascular disease.[108] More research is needed, including economic analyses, to determine the most beneficial strategies to pursue. As with reparatory health risks, risks of cardiovascular disease and stroke may be reduced in urban populations through filtration of ambient pollutants by tree cover.[109] Co-benefits of tree cover include heat-island alleviation, reduced energy use to cool buildings, and consequent reductions in greenhouse gas emissions.[110]

Fuel mixtures each have different particulate and other criteria pollutant profiles, and variously reduce net greenhouse gas emissions.[111] Fuel mixtures associated with high emissions of particulates or other pollutants such as nitrous oxides and carbon monoxide will have adverse impacts on cardiovascular health,[112] as these pollutants are associated with incidence of cardiovascular hospital admissions among those with existing heart disease.[113] Preliminary analysis of certain biodiesel blends is promising[114] but more research is needed to fully characterize likely health impacts of large-scale mitigation activities related to transport fuels.[115] Some biodiesel blends appear to produce emissions with few negative health consequences.[116] While an association between PM exposure and increased risk of cardiovascular disease has been demonstrated, it is unclear which chemical constituents mediate this effect. More research is needed to better identify these pollutants, which in turn will help to predict the potential benefits of alternative combustible fuels.[117] Due to

99   Suzuki, S, et al., American Heart Journal, 1997. 134(5): p. 974-977.
100 Leor, J, et al., New England Journal of Medicine, 1996. 334(7): p. 413-419.
101 Watanabe, H, et al., Journal of the American Medical Association, 2005. 294(3): p. 305-307.
102 Krousel-Wood, MA, et al., American Journal of the Medical Sciences, 2008. 336(2): p. 99-104.
103 Carod-Artal, FJ, Revista De Neurologia, 2007. 44(12): p. 755-763.
104 Ibid.
105 Bocchi, EA, et al., Heart, 2009. 95(3): p. 181-189.
106 Carcavallo, RU, Memorias Do Instituto Oswaldo Cruz, 1999. 94: p. 367-369.
107 Cox, J, et al., American Heart Journal, 1991. 122(5): p. 1449-1455.

108 Frumkin, H, et al., American Journal of Public Health, 2008. 98(3): p. 435-445.
109 Bowker, G, et al., Atmospheric Environment, 2007. 41: p. 8128-8139; Nowak, D, et al., Urban Forestry and Urban Greening, 2006. 4: p. 115-123.
110 Bolund, P, et al., Ecological Economics, 1999. 29: p. 293-301; McPherson, E, et al., Urban Ecosystems, 1997. 1: p. 49-61.
111 Hill, J, et al., Proc Natl Acad Sci U S A, 2006. 103(30): p. 11206-10.
112 Hill, J, et al., Proceedings of the National Academy of Sciences of the United States of America, 2009. 106(6): p. 2077-2082.
113 Mann, JK, et al., Environmental Health Perspectives, 2002. 110(12): p. 1247-1252.
114 McCormick, RL, Inhalation Toxicology, 2007. 19(12): p. 1033-1039.
115 Swanson, KJ, et al., Environmental Health Perspectives, 2007. 115(4): p. 496-499.
116 McCormick, RL, Inhalation Toxicology, 2007. 19(12): p. 1033-1039.
117 Brook, RD, et al., Circulation, 2004. 109(21): p. 2655-71.

the unique electrophysiological properties associated with the very high heart rates of the rodents most commonly used in researching dysrhythmia, these biomedical models do not always closely replicate human conditions. In contrast, the rates and underlying physiology of fish hearts are closer to humans and, as such, fish models should be explored as tools for understanding and screening the effects of various transport fuels. [118]

Projecting the health impacts of adaptation activities, particularly the increased use of air conditioning to protect vulnerable populations from extreme heat, requires assumptions regarding how these activities will be powered. For instance, if significant additional electricity demand is met through increased fossil fuel combustion, then there is likely to be increased exposure to particulates and ozone as a result. However, these exposures may be partially offset by the protective effect of air conditioning. Most other adaptation activities are likely to have little direct impact on cardiovascular disease incidence.

Research Needs

As noted, there are significant gaps in our understanding of climate change impacts on cardiovascular disease, particularly for morbidity, and there is virtually no research projecting future cardiovascular health impacts of climate change. Research needs include:

- increasing research on the incidence of cardiac dysrhythmias and associations with temperature and other environmental exposures

- enhancing research on the complex synergistic effect of temperature, weather variability, long-term climate change, and environmental exposures such as criteria air pollutants on the incidence of various cardiovascular disease outcomes

- intensifying investigation of the likely cardiovascular complications of VBZD prevalent in the United States and globally

- characterizing the multiple individual constituents of air pollution to better anticipate the health effects from switching the mix of pollutants in air through the use of alternative fuels

- studying strategies for incorporating cardiovascular disease outcomes in HIAs and integrated assessment climate models, including further characterization of exposure-outcome associations for cardiovascular morbidity in different geographic regions

- developing a national standard for heat-related mortality to facilitate epidemiologic study of mortality from heat and other co-morbid conditions [119]

- targeting research on early warning systems and health communications aimed at groups particularly at risk for adverse cardiovascular outcomes related to climate change

- identifying and quantifying the co-benefits to cardiovascular health of reducing our reliance on fossil fuel-based energy and changing emission scenarios

- characterizing both the potential health risks and benefits of novel fuels and other energy production activities being considered for large-scale adoption as part of a national mitigation strategy

Several cardiovascular disease research priorities dovetail with other areas. In particular, research into health impacts of increased temperature, extreme weather, and changes in air quality associated with climate change will inform research into cardiovascular health impacts. Similarly, research into early warning systems and integrated assessment models is transferable to other health outcomes associated with climate change, and research into the health impacts of potential mitigation and adaptation activities can be applied to other health outcomes sensitive to particulate and other emissions.

118   Milan, DJ, et al., Ibid.2009. 120(7): p. 553-9.

119   Wainwright, S, et al., American Journal of Epidemiology, 1994. 139(11): p. S49-S49.

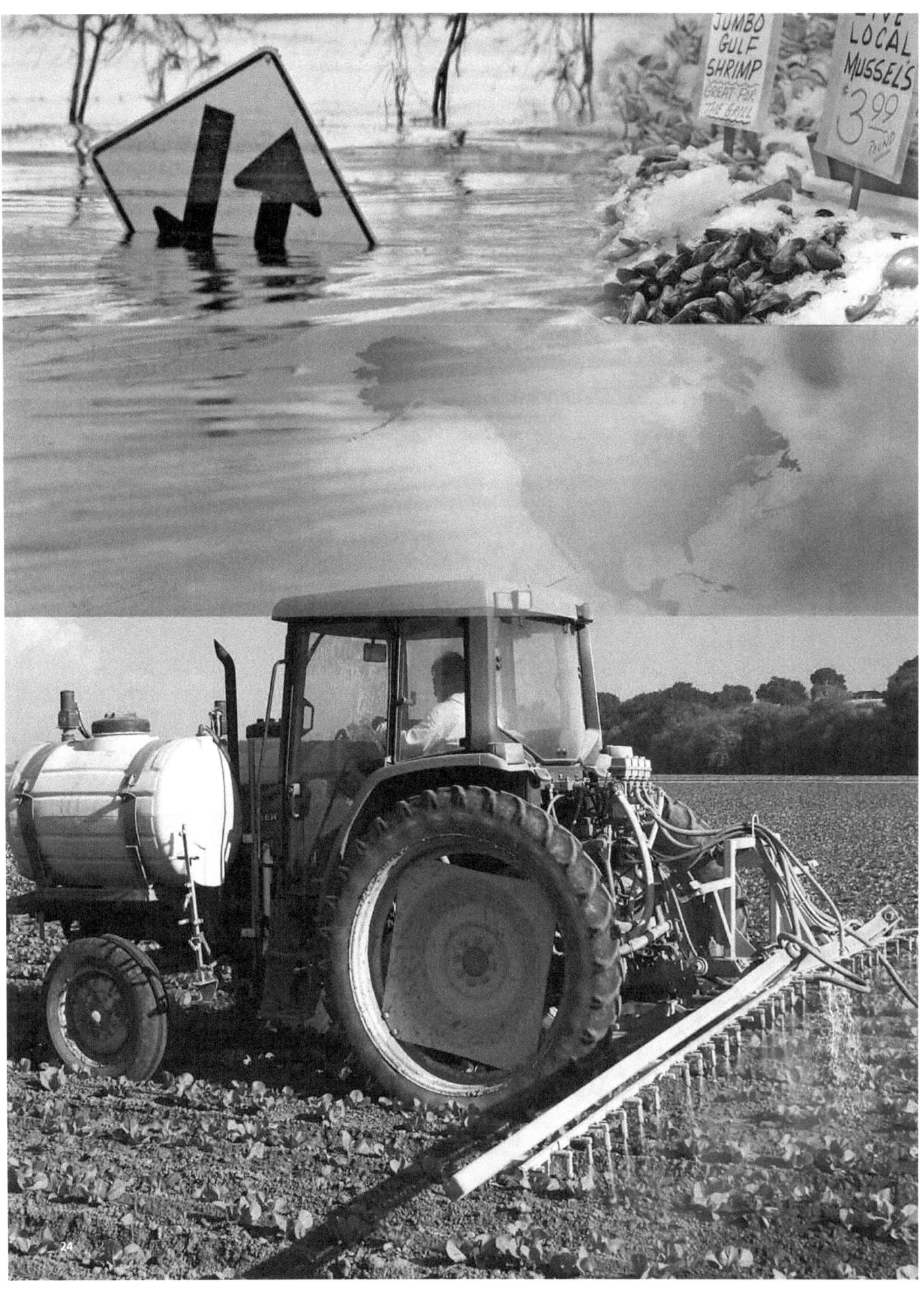

Foodborne Diseases and Nutrition

Nutrition is the sum of the processes by which humans and other living organisms take in food and use it for growth and nourishment. Along with clean air, water, and shelter, nutritious food is a basic necessity of life. Failure to obtain sufficient calories and an adequate mixture of macronutrients (calories, fat, proteins, carbohydrates), micronutrients (vitamins, minerals) and other bioactive components of food can result in illness and death. According to the United Nations Development Program, some 3.7 billion people worldwide are currently malnourished. While malnutrition and hunger are predominantly problems in the developing world, the United States and other developed countries still have significant populations affected by insufficient food resources and undernutrition.[120] Extreme weather events and changes in temperature and precipitation patterns can directly damage or destroy crops and other food supplies, as well as interrupt transport and distribution of food. This may happen seasonally, but is anticipated to become a more chronic problem under changing climate conditions. Indirectly, there is potential for harm from undernutrition or even famine resulting from damage to agricultural crops and related trade, economic, and social instability; diversion of staple crops for use in biofuels (corn for ethanol or other biofuels); changes in agricultural practices including those intended to mitigate or adapt to climate change; impaired ability to grow crops due to changing environmental conditions and water availability; and reduced availability and nutritional quality of protein from fisheries, aquaculture, and other marine-based foods.

In addition to being a source of essential nutrients, food can be a source of exposure for foodborne illness. Such illness results from ingesting food that is spoiled or contaminated with microbes, chemical residues such as pesticides, biotoxins, or other toxic substances. It is estimated that there are 38 million cases of foodborne illness in the United States each year, resulting in over 180,000 hospitalizations and 2,700 deaths.[121] Seafood contaminated with metals, biotoxins, toxicants, or pathogens; crops burdened with chemical pesticide residues or microbes; extreme shortages of staple foods; and malnutrition are among the possible effects of climate change on the production, quality, and availability of food.[122] The potential effects of climate change on foodborne illness, nutrition, and security are for the most part indirect

RESEARCH HIGHLIGHT

Climate change may impact rates of foodborne illness through increased temperatures, which are associated with increased incidence of foodborne gastroenteritis. Several species of *Vibrio*, naturally occurring marine bacteria, are sensitive to changes in ocean temperature. *Vibrio parahaemolyticus* infects oysters and is the leading cause of Vibrio-associated gastroenteritis in the United States.[1]

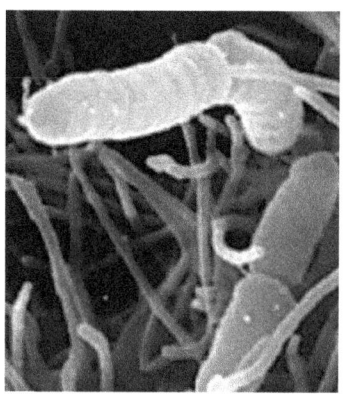

An outbreak in 2004 in Alaska has been linked to higher than normal ocean temperatures.[2] Other studies show a predictive relationship between sea surface temperature and *V. vulnificus* and *V. cholera*. Climate-driven changes in ocean temperature and coastal water quality are expected to increase the geographic range of these bacteria, and could be used to predict outbreaks. Increased temperatures also affect rates of other foodborne illnesses including campylobacteriosis and salmonellosis. A recent article examined the relationship between temperature and the weekly rates of several foodborne illnesses in England and Wales, including food poisoning, campylobacteriosis, and salmonellosis infections, and demonstrated this relationship. Research shows a significant correlation of these illnesses with ambient temperature at the time of illness and with the previous week's temperature.[3] Depending on the type of foodborne illness, for every degree centigrade rise in temperature, results showed 2.5–6% relative increase in the risk of foodborne illness. In the United States, good statistics on foodborne diseases are lacking, although estimates range from 6 million to 81 million illnesses and up to 9,000 deaths each year. Though current surveillance of foodborne illness in the United States is patchy and the burden of severe disease is not well known, further research may make it possible to translate these numbers into health impacts.

120 Nord, M., et al., Hosehold food security in the United States, 2008, ER Service, Editor: November, 2009, US Department of Agriculture: Washington, DC.

121 Mead, PS, et al., Emerg Infect Dis, 1999. 5(5): p. 607-25.

122 Intergovernmental Panel on Climate Change. Working Group II. 2007, Cambridge: Cambridge University Press. ix, 976 p.

1 US Food and Drug Administration, Quantitative risk assessment on the public health impact of pathogenic *Vibrio parahaemolyticus* in raw oysters. 2005.

2 McLaughlin, JB, et al., N Engl J Med, 2005. 353(14): p. 1463-70.

3 Lake, IR, et al., Epidemiol Infect, 2009. 137, p. 1538–1547.

and, in the United States at least, may be moderate and unlikely except in the event of disruption of government regulatory programs. However, on a global scale they are huge in terms of numbers of people likely to be affected and consequent human suffering. The Intergovernmental Panel on Climate Change projected with high confidence an increase in malnutrition and consequent disorders, including those related to child growth and development, as a result of climate change.[123] Some of these effects are already being felt in the wake of extreme weather events such as droughts, flooding, and hurricanes, and as such present a fairly immediate concern. The World Health Organization estimated that in 2000, there were over 77,000 deaths from malnutrition and 47,000 deaths from diarrhea (many from foodborne exposures) due to climate change.[124]

Impacts on Risks

The U.S. Climate Change Science Program (CCSP) reported a likely increase in the spread of several foodborne pathogens due to climate change, depending on the pathogens' survival, persistence, habitat range, and transmission in a changing environment.[125] Drought has been shown to encourage crop pests such as aphids, locusts, and whiteflies, as well as the spread of the mold *Aspergillus flavus* that produces aflatoxin, a substance that may contribute to the development of liver cancer in people who eat contaminated corn and nuts. Agronomists are also concerned that climate change-based increases in a variety of blasts, rusts, blights, and rots will further devastate already stressed crops, and thereby exacerbate malnutrition, poverty, and the need for human migration. The spread of agricultural pests and weeds may lead to the need for greater use of some toxic chemical herbicides, fungicides, and insecticides,[126] resulting in potential immediate hazards to farm workers and their families,[127] as well as longer-term hazards to consumers, particularly children.[128]

The safety of agricultural crops and fisheries also may be threatened through contamination with metals, chemicals, and other toxicants that may be released into the environment as a result of extreme weather events, particularly flooding, drought, and wildfires, due to climate change.[129] Global changes in ocean currents and water mass distribution, along with changes in Arctic ice cover, length of melt

season, hydrology, and precipitation patterns, will alter contaminant and pathogen pathways.[130] Contaminants include a wide range of chemicals and metals such as PCBs, PAHs, mercury, and cadmium; pharmaceuticals such as synthetic hormones, statins, and antibiotics; widely used industrial chemicals such as fire retardants, stain repellants, and non-stick coatings; and pesticides and herbicides for agricultural use and vector control for public health protection. The health effects of human exposure to these environmental agents via complex land and ocean food webs are not well documented or understood, but evidence from animal studies is showing that such compounds accumulate in foods at concentrations that may affect fetal development, immune function, and other biological processes. These agents often occur together and may act synergistically, producing potentially greater harm than a single agent.

Recent findings demonstrate that pathogens that can pose disease risks to humans occur widely in marine organisms and may be affected by climate change.[131] In one specific example, the CCSP noted the strong association between sea surface temperature and proliferation of many *Vibrio* bacteria species that occur naturally in the environment (including those that cause cholera), and suggested that rising temperatures would likely lead to increased occurrence of illness associated with *Vibrio* bacteria in the United States, especially seafood-borne disease associated with *V. vulnificus* and *V. parahaemolyticus*.[132] Rising temperatures and impacts on other environmental parameters such as ocean acidification may also lead to more virulent strains of existing pathogens and changes in their distribution, or the emergence of new pathogens.[133] Increased risks from animal-borne disease pathogens could be especially acute in human populations that are highly dependant on marine-based diets for subsistence and who live where environmental effects resulting from climate change are pronounced (for example in certain native populations in Alaska).[134] Increased acidity of water associated with climate change may alter environmental conditions leading to greater proliferation of microbes of a public health concern. This is a significant concern in molluscan shellfish, because ocean acidification may affect formation of their carbonate shells and immune responses, making them more vulnerable to microbial infection. The combined impact of potential contaminant-induced immune suppression and expanding ranges of disease-causing pathogens and biotoxins on food supply could be significant.

123. Ibid.
124. Campbell-Lendrum, D., et al. Environmental Burden of Disease Series, ed. A. Pruss-Ustun, et al. 2007, Geneva: World Health Organization. 66.
125. Gamble, JL, et al. 2008, Washington, D.C.: U.S. Climate Change Science Program. ix, 204 p.
126. Gregory, PJ, et al. J Exp Bot, 2009. 60(10): p. 2827-38.
127. Lynch, SM, et al., Environ Res, 2009. 109(7): p. 860-8, Park, SK, et al., Int J Occup Environ Health, 2009. 15(3): p. 274-81, Rusiecki, JA, et al., Environ Health Perspect, 2009. 117(4): p. 581-6.
128. Eskenazi, B, et al., Basic Clin Pharmacol Toxicol, 2008. 102(2): p. 228-36, Rosas, LG, et al., Curr Opin Pediatr, 2008. 20(2): p. 191-7.
129. Ebi, K, et al. In Analyses of the effects of global change on human health and welfare and human systems. A Report by the U.S. Climate Change Science Program and the Subcommittee on Global Change Research, J. Gamble, et al., Editors. 2008, USEPA: Washington, D. C.

130. Ibid.
131. Moore, SK, et al., Environmental Health: A Global Access Science Source, 2008. 7(SUPPL. 2).
132. Ebi, K, et al. In Analyses of the effects of global change on human health and welfare and human systems. A Report by the U.S. Climate Change Science Program and the Subcommittee on Global Change Research, J. Gamble, et al., Editors. 2008, USEPA: Washington, D. C.
133. Smolinski, MS, et al. 2003, Washington, D.C.: National Academies Press. xxviii, 367 p.
134. Sokurenko, EV, et al., Nat Rev Microbiol, 2006. 4(7): p. 548-55.

Mitigation and Adaptation

In the long term, mitigation and adaptation decisions affecting food and nutrition including, for example, the diversion of staple crops for biofuel feedstock, the increased need for agricultural chemicals due to climate-related increases in pests and changes in pest habitats, and planning needs for the maintenance of food supply infrastructure and transport in the wake of extreme weather events are important factors to be considered in a strategic research plan for climate change and health. The benefits of biofuels, genetically modified organisms, new pesticides, and alternative energy on nutrition and foodborne illness must also be considered. All of these technologies have great potential to help humans mitigate and adapt to climate change, and each should be carefully evaluated to ensure that the best are implemented.

Health implications, both positive and negative, of changes in animal agriculture and aquaculture as a result of climate change mitigation and adaptation need to be identified and quantified. For example, climate change events such as drought and flooding can result in changes in animal feed quality and the use of marginal lands for animal grazing affects water and habitat quality. Better understanding is needed of effects of the use of new or increased herbicides and pesticides in response to changes in growing conditions caused by climate change, as well as potential health effects for both humans and animals of ingestion of crops that have been genetically modified to withstand stress conditions caused by climate change. The health implications of biomass-based energy and biofuels, including interactions between climate mitigation strategies affecting agricultural and energy policies and availability of food, must be a priority area of research.

Research Needs

New efforts are needed to combine current and anticipated advances in detection and warning systems for food, nutrition, and foodborne health threats with epidemiologic studies on the occurrence and severity of poor nutrition and foodborne disease in humans. This is especially needed for high-risk populations such as women, infants, and children, and people in resource-constrained settings. Research needs include:

- projecting impacts of climate change including increases in CO_2, temperature, drought, floods, and other extreme weather events, and changes in growing seasons on food production, availability, contamination, and nutritional value

- understanding and predicting potential ecosystem changes from climate change that may establish new foodborne pathogens, chemical contaminants, or biotoxins, as well as new pathways for human exposure

- assessing the impacts of climate change on outbreak incidence, geographic range, and growth cycles of insect pests and pathogens that can infect food crops and seafood, and cause human disease

- understanding the effects of changes in food safety due to climate change-related alterations in the accumulation and toxicity of foodborne contaminants, biotoxins, and pathogens

- understanding of changes in nutritional status associated with climate change that may increase individual susceptibility to the adverse health impacts of other environmental exposures such as chemicals and heavy metals

- improving surveillance of disease-causing agents (chemical contaminants, pathogens, toxins) in food animals, agricultural crops, and seafood, as well as monitoring of exposed human populations in order to improve estimates of disease related to contamination of the food supply

- identifying and characterizing aspects of food production and distribution systems that will reduce risk of contamination and disease and ensure sustainability under climate change scenarios

- understanding the effect of ocean acidification from climate change-related increases in air pollution on seafood quality and availability

- developing and implementing models linking climate change and other environmental data (such as land use, land cover, hydrology) to crops and seafood to improve prediction and risk assessment

- developing and implementing early warning systems to manage agriculture and fisheries risks related to climate change, including improved communications with domestic and international food security agencies

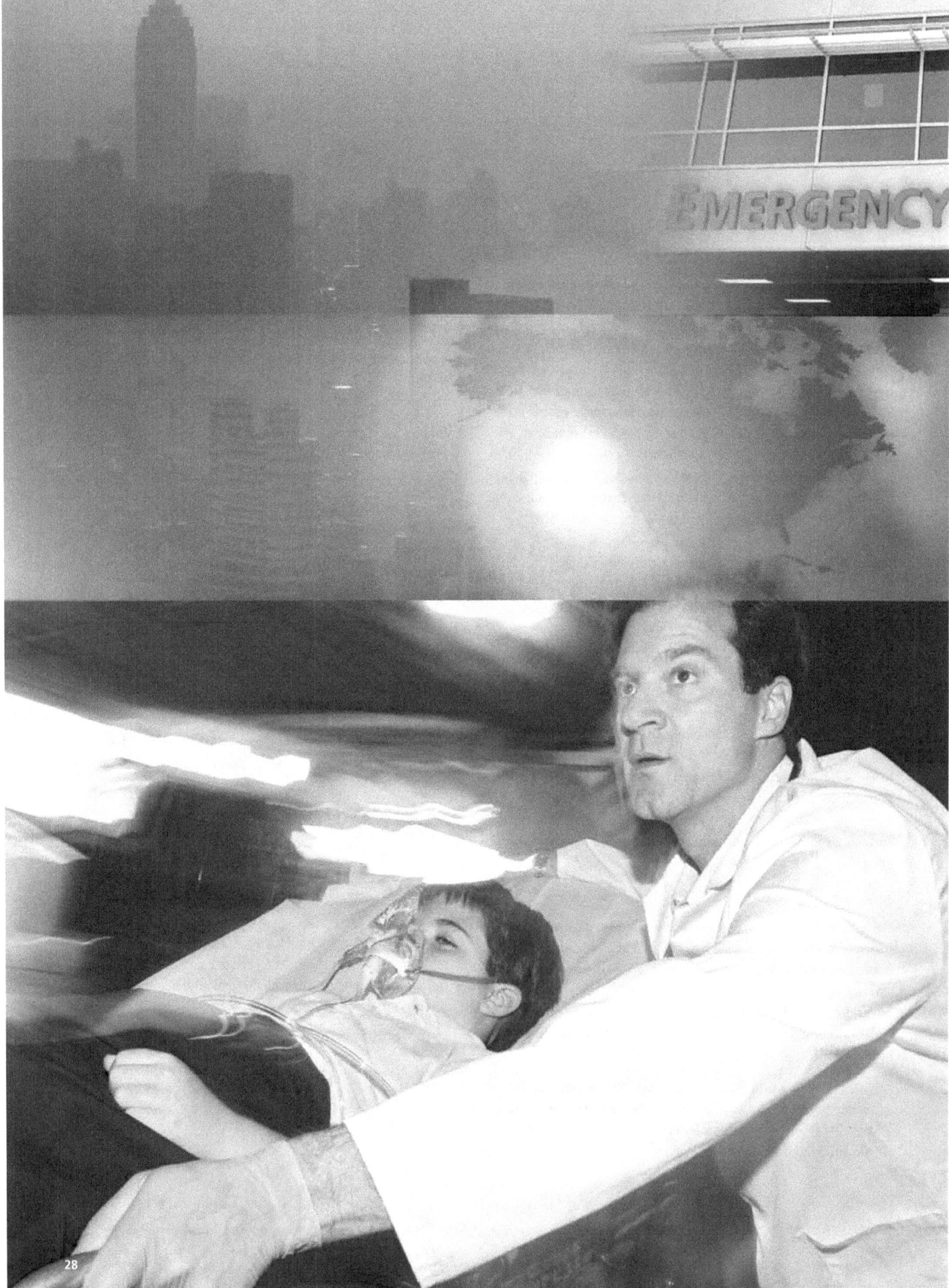

Heat-Related Morbidity and Mortality

As a result of anthropogenic climate change, global mean temperatures are rising, and are expected to continue to increase regardless of progress in reducing greenhouse emissions.[135] Global average temperatures are projected to increase between 1.8 and 4.0°C by end of this century.[136] Climate change is expected to raise overall temperature distribution and contribute to an increase in the frequency of extreme heat events, or heat waves.[137] Temperature, particularly temperature extremes, is associated with a wide range of health impacts.

The health outcomes of prolonged heat exposure include heat exhaustion, heat cramps, heat stroke, and death.[138] Extreme heat events cause more deaths annually in the United States than all other extreme weather events combined.[139] In the United States, an average of 688 persons succumb to heat-related death per year.[140] Prolonged exposure to heat may also result in additional illness and death by exacerbating preexisting chronic conditions such as various respiratory, cerebral, and cardiovascular diseases,[141] as well as increasing risk for patients taking psychotropic drug treatment for mental disorders,[142] due to the body's impaired ability to regulate temperature. Figures for these illnesses and deaths may be dramatically underestimated as disparities in health care make morbidity measurements difficult and heat is rarely identified as an official cause of death. Some public health response organizations are in the process of developing heat early warning systems for anticipated heat wave events and extended warm periods.

Varying age groups have been shown to be sensitive to all-cause mortality under excessive heat stress, including adults over 65, children, and infants under 1 year of age.[143] For type-specific mortality, sensitivity to death from respiratory disease has been demonstrated in the general population and in the elderly.[144] In general, risk of respiratory death due to heat stress is greater than that of cardiovascular effects. Sensitivity to cerebrovascular disease-related death has been reported in Europe.[145] More commonly, sensitivity to cardiovascular disease-related mortality associated with heat has been seen in the whole population, as well as among the elderly. Elevated hyperthermia death risk also has been seen among the elderly in the United States.[146] However, heat-related risks are not regionally or locally uniform; demographic shifts in the United States will produce concentrations of larger populations with higher mean age, and thereby, heightened vulnerability to excessive heat.[147]

Impacts on Risk

Both increased average temperatures and increasingly frequent and severe extreme heat events produce increased risks of heat-related illness and death that can be significant: the European heat wave of 2003 caused more than 35,000 excess deaths.[148] Human susceptibility to heat-related illness depends on several different factors, from physiologic adaptation to the local environment to socioeconomic status, and the impact of these changing exposures will depend on the vulnerability of exposed populations. As noted above, host factors such as age and the burden of other serious illnesses such as heart disease and diabetes that might exacerbate heat-related problems are important. In the United States, the number of individuals 65 years of age and older (who are more susceptible to heat effects) is expected to increase from 12.4% in 2000 to 20% in 2060.[149] Socioeconomic factors also determine vulnerability; economically disadvantaged and socially isolated people face higher burdens of death from heat.[150]

Cities and climate are co-evolving in a manner that will certainly amplify both the health effects of heat and the vulnerability of urban populations to heat-related deaths by magnifying the increased temperatures caused by climate change as compared to adjacent rural and suburban locales.[151,152] The urban built environment can

135 Houghton, JT, et al. 2001. Cambridge ; New York: Cambridge University Press. x, 881 p.
136 Intergovernmental Panel on Climate Change. Working Group II. 2007. Cambridge: Cambridge University Press. ix, 976 p.
137 Meehl, GA, et al., Science, 2004. 305(5686): p. 994-7.
138 Ellis, FP, Trans R Soc Trop Med Hyg, 1976. 70(5-6): p. 402-11.; Kilbourne, EM, et al., JAMA, 1982. 247(24): p. 3332-6.
139 Luber, G, et al., Am J Prev Med, 2008. 35(5): p. 429-35.
140 Merchandani, H, et al., Journal of the American Medical Association, 1993. 270(7): p. 610-810.
141 Kovats, RS, et al., Heat stress and public health: A critical review, in Annual Review of Public Health. 2008. p. 41-55.
142 Davido, A, et al., Emerg Med J, 2006. 23(7): p. 515-8.
143 Bytomski, JR, et al., Curr Sports Med Rep, 2003. 2(6): p. 320-4; Piver, WT, et al., Environ Health Perspect, 1999. 107(11): p. 911-6; Ye, F, et al., Environ Health Perspect, 2001. 109(4): p. 355-9; Curriero, FC, et al., Am J Epidemiol, 2002. 155(1): p. 80-7; Davis, RE, et al., Environmental Health Perspectives, 2003. 111(14): p. 1712-1718; Gosling, SN, et al., Climatic Change, 2009. 92(3-4): p. 299-341.
144 Kovats, RS, et al., Heat stress and public health: A critical review, in Annual Review of Public Health. 2008. p. 41-55.

145 Gosling, SN, et al., Climatic Change, 2009. 92(3-4): p. 299-341.
146 Curriero, FC, et al., Am J Epidemiol, 2002. 155(1): p. 80-7.
147 Luber, G, et al., Am J Prev Med, 2008. 35(5): p. 429-35.
148 Vandentorren, S, et al., Am J Public Health, 2004. 94(9): p. 1518-20.
149 Wilmoth, JM, et al., Research on Aging, 2006. 28(3): p. 269-288.
150 Gosling, SN, et al., Climatic Change, 2009. 92(3-4): p. 299-341.
151 Brazel, AJ, et al. in Encyclopedia of world climatology, JE Oliver, Editor. 2005, Springer: Dordrecht, The Netherlands. XX, 854 p.
152 Patz, JA, et al., Nature, 2005. 438(7066): p. 310-7.

both exacerbate and alleviate the effects of heat. For example, high concentrations of buildings in urban areas cause what is known as the urban heat island effect: generating as well as absorbing and releasing heat, resulting in urban centers that are several degrees warmer than surrounding areas. Expanding parks and green spaces and increasing the density of trees in and around cities can help to reduce this effect.[153] It is estimated that 60% of the global population will live in cities by 2030, greatly increasing the total human population exposed to extreme heat.[154]

Researchers comparing annual heat-related deaths for the city of Los Angeles in the 1990s to those projected for the mid- and late-21st century have concluded that heat-related deaths will increase, perhaps up to seven-fold.[155] Another study assessing 21 U.S. cities estimates that for most of the cities, summer deaths will increase dramatically and winter deaths will decrease slightly, even with acclimatization. This shift to higher summer heat-related deaths will likely outweigh the extra winter deaths averted.[156] Climate change is projected to increase the average number of summer-time heat-related deaths, with the greatest increases occurring in mid-latitude major cities where summer climate variability is greatest. Noting that the number of current heat-related deaths in U.S. cities is considerable in spite of mortality displacement (reduced mortality in the months following a heat event due to increased early deaths of critically ill people who would have died in the near-term regardless) and the increased use of air conditioning, a substantial rise in weather-related deaths is the most likely direct health outcome of climate change.[157]

It is difficult to make valid projections of heat-related illness and death under varying climate change scenarios. A review of past changes in heat-related deaths found few significant relationships for any decade or demographic group, and suggested that improved medical care, air conditioning use, and other adaptation efforts were the causes of reduced death, stating that despite increasing stressful weather events, heat–related deaths are preventable, as evidenced by the decline of all-cause mortality during heat events over the past 35 years.[158] Overall, research suggests that under a climate change scenario using current anthropogenic emissions

trends, there will be a small increase in the overall U.S. heat-related death rate by the end of the 21st century.[159] A standardized definition and methodology for identifying heat-related health outcomes is needed for surveillance and to evaluate temperature-related illness and death.

Mitigation and Adaptation

While climate change is likely to increase the burden of heat-related illness and death in the United States, many of these outcomes are preventable. With aggressive public health actions and widespread physiologic and behavioral adaptations such as robust heat early warning systems and other health communications, increased air conditioning use, decreased time spent outdoors, and increased wearing of sun-shielding clothing it will be possible to reduce overall rates of illness and death, though some of these measures may result in negative health consequences as well.[160]

Adaptation occurs through a range of physiological, behavioral, and technological mechanisms, and the slight reduction in heat-related deaths in the United States, despite warming trends, is likely a result of adaptation. In a report on acclimatization in elderly people over time, researchers showed both a declining risk of heat-related cardiovascular deaths until no excess risk remained and a steady risk of cold-related deaths.[161] This effect was observed in other populations as well: over four 10-year time periods in the 20th century in London, progressive reductions in temperature-related deaths (both cold and hot) were reported, despite an aging population.[162] Cities with cooler climates tend to experience more heat-related deaths than those with warmer climates because populations can acclimatize to some extent to heat and because populations in warmer climates are more likely to have access to air conditioning. Heat-related death rates declined significantly over four decades (the period of 1964–1998) in 19 of 28 U.S. metropolitan areas[163] although the trend seems to have leveled off since the 1990s.[164]

Although air conditioning may explain the reduced heat-related death risk, it also may be due to improved standards of living, better access to medical care, biophysical coping mechanisms, and infrastructural adaptations. Depending on methods of power generation and the air conditioning technology used, however,

153 Bolund, P. et al., Ecological Economics, 1999. 29: p. 293-301; McPherson, E. et al., Urban Ecosystems, 1997. 1: p 49-61.
154 United Nations Department of Economic and Social Affairs Population Division World Urbanization Prospects: The 2005 Revision, PD United Nations Department of Economic and Social Affairs, Editor. 2006, United Nations Department of Economic and Social Affairs, Population Division: Geneva.
155 Hayhoe, K. et al., Proc Natl Acad Sci U S A, 2004. 101(34): p. 12422-7.
156 McMichael, AJ, et al., Lancet, 2006. 367(9513): p. 859-869.
157 Kalkstein, LS, et al., Environ Health Perspect, 1997. 105(1): p. 84-93.
158 Davis, RE, et al., Climate Research, 2002. 22(2): p. 175-184.

159 Deschenes, O. et al., Climate Change, Mortality, and Adaptation: Evidence from Annual Fluctuations in Weather in the US, in Center for the Study of Energy Markets Paper. 2007, Center for the Study of Energy Markets: Santa Barbara, CA. p. 61.
160 McGeehin, MA, et al., Environ Health Perspect, 2001. 109 Suppl 2: p. 185-9.
161 Barnett, AG, Epidemiology, 2007. 18(3): p. 369-72.
162 Carson, C, et al., Am J Epidemiol, 2006. 164(1): p. 77-84.
163 Davis, RE, et al., Environmental Health Perspectives, 2003. 111(14): p. 1712-1718.
164 Sheridan, SC, et al., Natural Hazards, 2009. 50(1): p. 145-160.

increased use of air conditioning may result in higher greenhouse gas emissions.[165] In addition, to the extent that power grids become overburdened during excessive heat events, resulting blackouts and brownouts could leave populations at increased risk of deaths.

From a public health perspective, proactive heat wave response plans may prove to be a more sustainable adaptation strategy. Following a 2003 heat wave in Western Europe, France established a National Heat Plan incorporating several preventive measures aimed at reducing the risks related to high temperatures including a heat early warning system. During a lasting and severe heat wave in 2006, the excess death rate in France was much lower than expected given the high numbers of deaths three years earlier; research suggests that the decrease may have resulted from implementation of this plan.[166]

Research Needs

Research needs to improve understanding of heat-related illness and death, as well as impacts of heat mitigation and adaptation, include:

- developing and implementing a standard definition of heat-related health outcomes, as well as standard methodologies for surveillance of outcomes and evaluation of adaptations

- understanding risk factors for illness and death associated with both acute exposure to extreme heat events and long-term, chronic exposure to increased average temperatures, including how such exposure may alter human physiology (for example, by impacting the body's ability to metabolize and excrete harmful environmental toxicants)

- identifying which temperature-related metrics are most strongly related to increased hospitalization and mortality during heat waves

- quantifying the combined effects of exposure to heat waves and ambient air pollution on excessive illness and death

- conducting comparative analyses of heat-related death risks for application to national scale analyses

- determining attributes of communities, including regional and seasonal differences, that are more resilient or vulnerable to adverse health impacts from heat waves

- assessing the health benefits of the use of environmental design principles to reduce the high thermal mass of urban areas

- characterizing the likelihood and nature of multi-system failures, such as power grid failure, that could lead to significant morbidity and mortality during a heat wave

- enhancing the ability of current climate models to capture the observed frequency and intensity of heat waves across various timescales to support weather-climate predictions and use of heat early warning systems in decision making

- evaluating heat response plans, focusing on environmental risk factors, identification of high-risk populations, effective communications strategies, and rigorous methods for evaluating effectiveness on the local level

165 Yoshida, Y, Carbon Balance Manag, 2006. 1: p. 12.
166 Fouillet, A, et al., Int J Epidemiol, 2008. 37(2): p. 309-17.

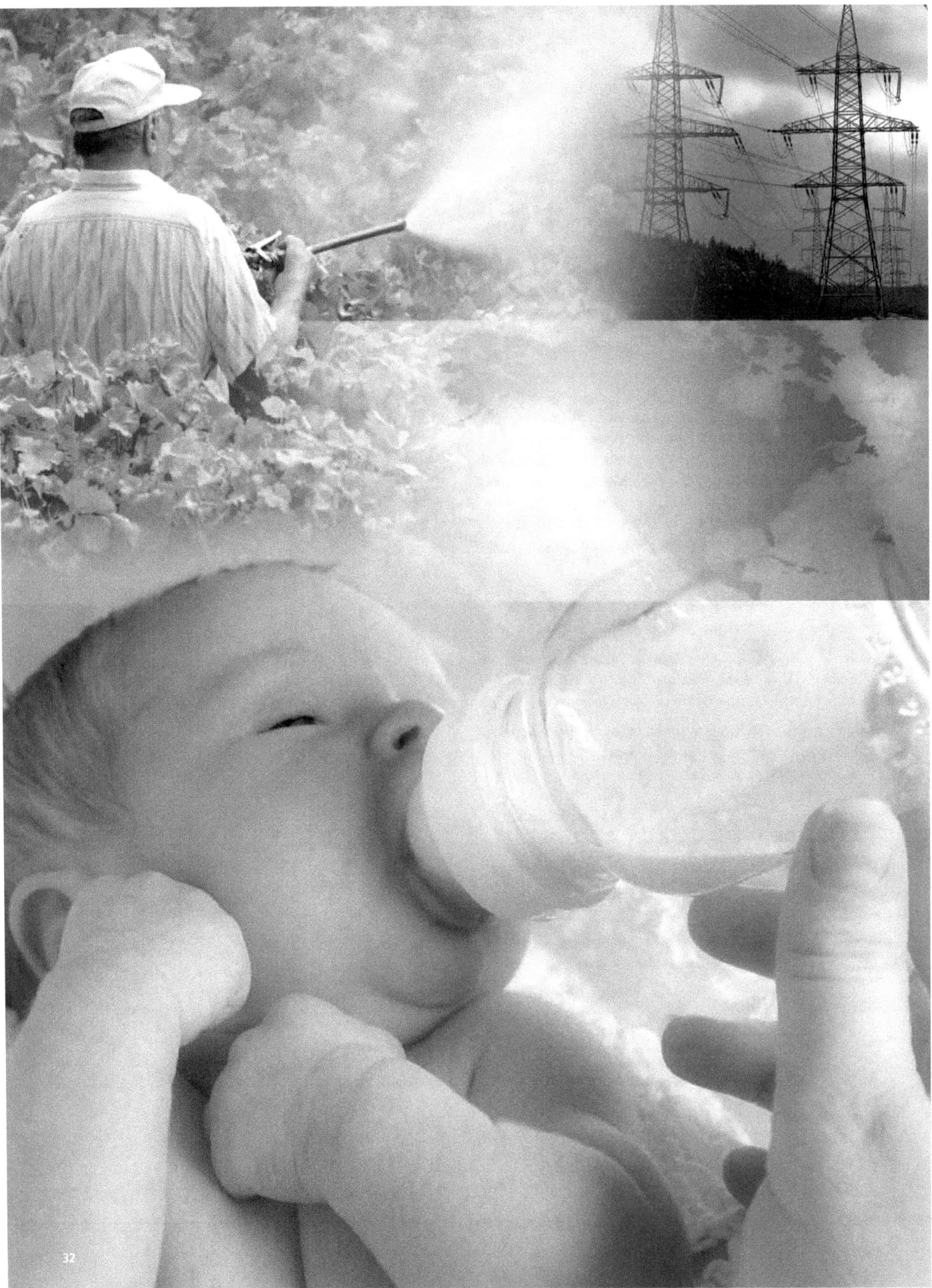

Human Development

Most humans develop in a predictable fashion, growing from a fertilized egg to fetus, newborn, toddler, child, adolescent, and adult in a way that is fairly well understood. The environment can be a potent modifier of normal development and behavior. Environmental effects on development include subtle changes such as small reductions in IQ from exposure to lead,[167] changes in onset of puberty from exposure to endocrine disrupting chemicals,[168] birth defects such as cleft palate due to dioxin-like compounds,[169] and fetal loss through exposure-related spontaneous abortion.[170] According to the Centers for Disease Control and Prevention, about 3% of all children born in the United States have a birth defect, some of which can be attributed to environmental causes. Birth defects are a leading cause of death in children, accounting for almost 20% of all infant deaths. Babies born with birth defects also have a greater chance of illness and long-term disability than children without birth defects.[171] Some of these birth defects have been steadily increasing over the last 20 years, for example the rates of congenital heart defects have doubled,[172] suggesting a possible environmental linkage, although other explanations such as better reporting may also explain the rise.

Recent research into early functional programming has opened a new perspective on the developmental and early life origins of human disease.[173] Vulnerable periods during human development include preconception (gametogenesis), preimplantation, the fetal period, and early childhood. Environmental exposures during these periods can lead to functional deficits and developmental changes through several mechanisms including genetic mutations and epigenetic change. Some chemicals damage DNA directly, causing mutations in gametes or the developing fetus that can lead to later disease or conditions that increase disease risks such as obesity.[174] For example, toxins such as domoic acid, a biotoxin released from harmful algal blooms and taken up by seafood and

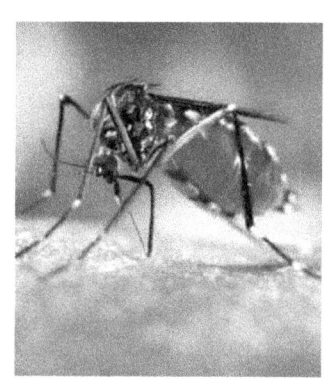

RESEARCH HIGHLIGHT

Many of the chemicals that we use to control pests and improve crop yields can impact human development. Climate change will alter rainfall and temperature in various parts of the planet. In some cases, climate change will lead to changes in agricultural practices for crop yields that might increase pesticide use and thereby increase human exposures. Changes in the range of mosquitoes and other pests that can carry disease also may lead to an increase in the use of legacy pesticides (e.g. DDT). Malaria is rare in the United States, although the number of cases (imported or indigenous) have been increasing over the last decade in some locations.[1] The insecticide DDT is highly efficient for the control of mosquitoes that are capable of transmitting malaria to humans. Although withdrawn from use in the United States, DDT is still used as a desperate expedient to control mosquitoes in malaria-endemic areas around the world. DDT and its principal metabolite, DDE, are persistent in the environment and in humans. Research has shown that women whose mothers had high DDT levels in their blood when they were *in utero* have shortened menstrual cycles and a reduced chance of getting pregnant. A landmark study showed that for every 10 milligrams per liter of DDT in mother's serum, the probability of pregnancy for the daughter dropped by 32%.[2] Other pesticides also have been linked to similar decreases in fertility.[3] Later studies on similar exposures showed equivocal results on time-to-pregnancy, but suggested effects on fetal loss, child growth, and male reproductive development.[4]

167 Stein, J., et al., J Dev Behav Pediatr, 2002. 23(1 Suppl): p. S13-22.
168 Rogan, WJ, et al., Int J Hyg Environ Health, 2007. 210(5): p. 659-67.
169 Pradat, P, et al., Birth Defects Res A Clin Mol Teratol, 2003. 67(12): p. 968-70.
170 Bukowski, JA, Regul Toxicol Pharmacol, 2001. 33(2): p. 147-56.
171 CDC. Birth Defects, 2009 [cited 2009 July 22]; Available from: http://www.cdc.gov/ncbddd/bd/.
172 Correa-Villaseñor A, et al., Birth Defects Res A Clin Mol Teratol, 2003. 67(9): p. 617-24
173 Aagaard-Tillery, KM, et al., Journal of Molecular Endocrinology, 2008. 41(2): p. 91-102.
174 Wadhwa, PD, et al., Semin Reprod Med, 2009. 27(5): p. 358-68.

1 WHO. Global Malaria Programme. 2008, Geneva: World Health Organization. xx, 190 p.
2 Cohn, BA, et al., Lancet, 2003. 361(9376): p. 2205-6.
3 Roeleveld, N, et al., Curr Opin Obstet Gynecol, 2008. 20(3): p. 229-33.
4 Longnecker, MP, et al., Am J Epidemiol, 2002. 155(4): p. 313-22, Law, DC, et al., Am J Epidemiol, 2005. 162(6): p. 523-32, Longnecker, MP, et al., Environ Res, 2005. 97(2): p. 127-33, Ribas-Fito, N, et al., Int J Epidemiol, 2006. 35(4): p. 853-8.

marine mammals, can bioaccumulate in amniotic fluid and alter fetal development.[175] Chemicals can also cause epigenetic changes that alter the way DNA is interpreted, leading to inheritable functional changes without changing DNA itself. These epigenetic changes could have consequences for many diseases and developmental changes.[176] For example, maternal undernutrition may act on the developing fetus to program the risks for adverse health outcomes such as cardiovascular disease, obesity, and metabolic syndrome in adult life. In this way, changes in maternal nutrition and *in utero* exposure to certain chemicals or biotoxins due to climate change may impact the health of future generations through epigenetic changes before conception and during pregnancy. Developmental changes can result in a lifetime of suffering and have significant societal costs in terms of resources, medical care, and lost productivity.[177]

Impacts on Risk

People at different stages of life can respond very differently to environmental changes. Some changes to the environment resulting from climate change could alter normal human development both in the womb and later in life. Foodborne illness and food insecurity, both likely outcomes of climate change [see chapter on Nutrition and Foodborne Diseases], may lead to malnutrition. While adult humans exposed to mild famine usually recover quite well when food again becomes plentiful, nutritional reductions to a fetus in the womb appear to have lasting effects throughout life.[178] Malnutrition and undernutrition in pregnant women are a global cause of low birth weight and other poor birth outcomes that are associated with later developmental deficits. Malnutrition is predominantly a problem in the developing world, but in the United States, one in six children still live in poverty,[179] and other developed countries also have substantial populations with insufficient food resources and undernutrition[180] that could be made worse by climate change. Climate change effects on food availability and nutritional content could have a marked, multigenerational effect on human development.[181]

Changes in patterns and concentrations of contaminants entering the marine environment due to climate change will impact seafood species, many of which provide a major source of protein to global populations. Such contaminants, particularly metals such as mercury and lead that accumulate in fish and seafood, are a special

concern for human developmental effects.[182] Similarly, an increase in the use of herbicides and pesticides for agricultural purposes, as well as alterations in environmental degradation of such chemicals due to changes in climate, could result in increased exposures that would exceed safety guidelines and increase the risk of developmental changes.[183]

Other environmental exposures to pregnant women and to children that areassociated with climate change also present hazards to normal human development. For example, certain commercial chemicals present in storage sites or hazardous waste sites can alter human development. Flooding from extreme weather events and sea-level rise are likely to result in the release of some of these chemicals and heavy metals, most likely affecting drinking and recreational waters. Some of these, including mercury and lead, have known negative developmental effects.

And while more research is required, there is good reason for concern based on our current body of knowledge of certain toxic metals and persistent organic compounds. Of the metals likely to become more prevalent in human environments due to climate change, inorganic arsenic is of great concern because it is a potent human carcinogen, it alters the immune system, and it is a general poison that is lethal at certain doses. More than 100 million people worldwide are exposed to arsenic through groundwater contamination and industrial emissions. Both inorganic and methylated forms of arsenic have been shown to impede fetal development and increase spontaneous abortions.[184] Persistent organic compounds, even those no longer in use in many locales such as DDT and PCBs, could increase in some human environments and decrease in others as a result of flooding and extreme weather events due to climate change[185] Many of the Superfund toxic waste sites in the United States contain PCBs and dioxins that have been linked to cognitive deficits in children that continue throughout their lives. It is expected that every person on the planet carries some body burden of PCBs, but people living near contaminated sites have greater exposures and an increased risk of disease.[186] Dioxins, PCBs, asbestos, benzene, flame retardants, certain pesticides, and other chemicals are known to be immunotoxicants. Changes to the immune system during development can remain throughout life, possibly resulting in a reduced capacity to fight serious infection and an increased risk of several other diseases including cancer.

175 Maucher, JM, et al., Environmental Health Perspectives, 2007. 115(12): p. 1743-1746.
176 Mathers, JC, Nutrigenomics - Opportunities in Asia, 2007. 60: p. 42-48.
177 CDC. Birth Defects, 2009 [cited 2009 July 22]; Available from: http://www.cdc.gov/ncbddd/bd/.
178 Mathers, JC, Nutrigenomics - Opportunities in Asia, 2007. 60: p. 42-48.
179 Nord, M, et al., Hosehold food security in the United States, 2008, ER Service, Editor. November, 2009, US Department of Agriculture: Washington, DC.
180 Nord, M, et al., Hosehold food security in the United States, 2008, ER Service, Editor. November, 2009, US Department of Agriculture: Washington, DC.
181 Noyes, PD, et al., Environment International, 2009. 35(6): p. 971-986.

182 Booth, S, et al., Environ Health Perspect, 2005. 113(5): p. 521-6.
183 Macdonald, RW, et al., Human and Ecological Risk Assessment, 2003. 9(3): p. 643-660.
184 Tofail, F, et al., Environmental Health Perspectives, 2009. 117(2): p. 288-293.
185 Macdonald, RW, et al., Human and Ecological Risk Assessment, 2003. 9(3): p. 643-660, Macdonald, RW, et al., Sci Total Environ, 2005. 342(1-3): p. 5-86.
186 Franzblau, A, et al., Chemosphere, 2009. 74(3): p. 395-403.

Climate change may alter the abundance and distribution of harmful algal blooms and their associated biotoxin accumulation in fish and seafood.[187] Currently there are over 100 known biotoxins associated with harmful algal blooms, and the biological effects of most are currently unknown; however, some have been shown to cross the placenta and affect the developing fetus.[188] It is partly for this reason though that fish species provide excellent biomedical models for developmental toxicity research, particularly the study of congenital heart defects. Such defects are notoriously difficult to study in standard rodent models due to the early dependency of mammalian embryos on circulatory function to provide oxygen. Because fish embryos are not dependent on early circulation for oxygen, fish models have made highly significant contributions to cardiac developmental studies in the past decade.[189]

Mitigation and Adaptation

In regions where water availability is a growing concern, there will be an increasing need to reuse water or seek alternate sources of water that may be of lower quality. This may result in new treatment options that may require the use of additional or more toxic chemicals.

Changes in energy source policies also could increase exposures to numerous airborne metal particulates, many of which, such as lead, have known adverse developmental impacts.[190] Given the large number of chemicals that are currently in commerce, the unknown degree to which climate change will alter human exposure to these compounds, and the lack of data on the developmental toxicity of most of these compounds, this is an area strongly in need of additional research.

Access to prenatal health care and to early intervention services is critical in preventing and mitigating birth defects and impacts on human development. Following extreme weather events, such health care and services potentially may be disrupted for extended periods of time, increasing the risk of adverse long-term consequences for mothers, children, and society.

Research Needs

Research is needed to evaluate climate-related impacts at different life stages including direct and epigenetic effects (through exposures to mothers and fathers) that may be hazardous to human development. Such research could improve understanding of the long-term effects on human development and provide guidance on how mitigation and adaptation can reduce this health burden. Research needs include:

- understanding the effects of climate change-induced stress on human reproduction and development, including chronic and acute heat stress, and traumatic stress as a result of extreme weather events

- understanding how malnutrition may alter human development, how climate change may exacerbate such alterations, and how to develop effective strategies to minimize these impacts in vulnerable populations

- understanding the impacts of changes in weather patterns and ecosystems on the incidence, exposure, and distribution of chemical contaminants and biotoxins known to cause developmental disorders

- expanding the use of marine species as biomedical models and sentinels for understanding effects of contaminants and biotoxins on human reproduction and development

- understanding the implications of mitigation strategies, including changes in energy policies and new technologies, on the production, use, and storage of heavy metals and chemicals that are known to cause developmental disorders

- understanding how weather events affect access to health care and the implications of this for normal human development

187 Niemi, G. et al., Environmental Health Perspectives, 2004. 112(9): p. 979-986.
188 Ibid.
189 Chico, TJ, et al., Trends Cardiovasc Med, 2008. 18(4): p. 150-5.
190 Gohlke, JM, et al., Environmental Health Perspectives, 2008. 116(6): p. A236-A237.

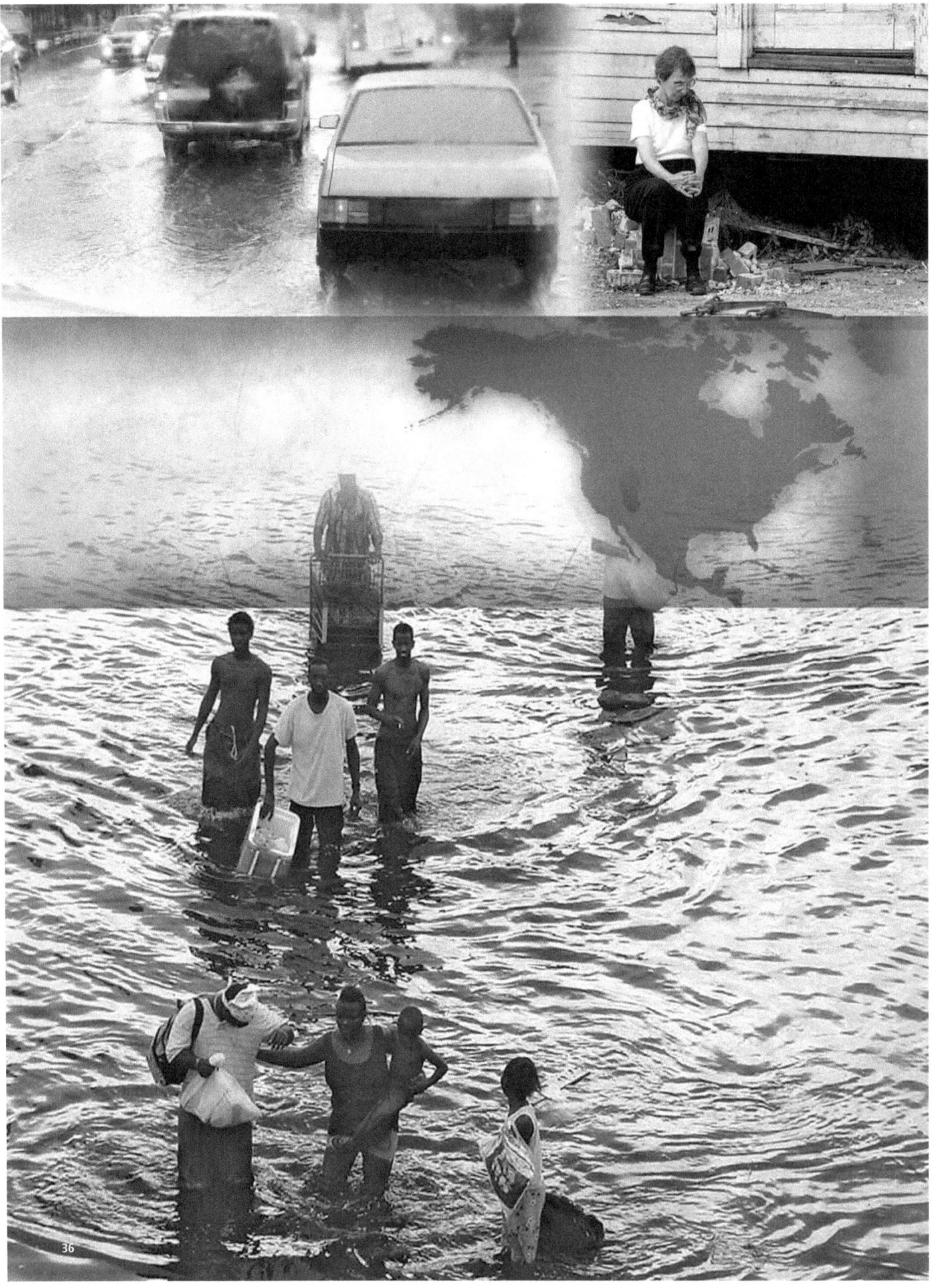

Mental Health and Stress-Related Disorders

Mental health disorders comprise a broad class of illnesses from mild disorders, such as social phobias and fear of speaking in public, to severe diseases including depression and suicidal ideation. Many mental health disorders can also lead to other chronic diseases and even death. Stress-related disorders derive from abnormal responses to acute or prolonged anxiety, and include diseases such as obsessive-compulsive disorder and post-traumatic stress disorder. It is estimated that 26.2% of Americans over the age of 18 suffer from a diagnosable mental health disorder in a given year; 9.5% suffer from mood disorders, and 6% suffer from serious mental illness.[191] However, mental health is an area of public health that is often a low research priority and one whose impacts on human and societal well being are typically underestimated, both within the United States and globally. It also is an area of public health in which disparities exist among socioeconomic groups in both access to and quality of care and treatment.[192]

Psychological impacts of climate change, ranging from mild stress responses to chronic stress or other mental health disorders, are generally indirect and have only recently been considered among the collection of health impacts of climate change.[193] Mental health concerns are among some of the most potentially devastating effects in terms of human suffering, and among the most difficult to quantify and address. A variety of psychological impacts can be associated with extreme weather and other climate related events. There has been significant research conducted depicting ways in which extreme weather events can lead to mental health disorders associated with loss, social disruption, and displacement, as well as cumulative effects from repeated exposure to natural disasters.[194] The effects of climate change impact the social, economic, and environmental determinants of mental health, with the most severe consequences being felt by communities who were already disadvantaged prior to the event.[195] Extreme weather events such as hurricanes, wildfires, and flooding, can create increased anxiety and emotional stress about the future,[196] as well as create added stress to vulnerable communities already experiencing social, economic, and environmental disruption. Individuals already vulnerable to mental health disease and stress-related disorders are likely to be at increased risk of exacerbated effects following extreme weather or other climate change events. Prolonged heat and cold events can create chronic stress situations that may initiate or exacerbate health problems in populations already suffering from mental disease and stress-related disorders. In addition, psychotropic drugs interfere with the body's ability to regulate temperature; individuals being treated with these drugs could be at increased risk of heat-related illness during extreme heat events.[197]

The severity of mental health impacts following an extreme climate event will depend on the degree to which there is sufficient coping and support capacity, both during and following the event.[198] During the recovery period following an extreme event, mental health problems and stress-related disorders can arise from geographic displacement, damage or loss of property, death or injury of loved ones, and the stress involved with recovery efforts.[199] The most common mental health conditions associated with extreme events range from acute traumatic stress to more chronic stress-related conditions such as post-traumatic stress disorder, complicated grief, depression, anxiety disorders, somatic complaints, poor concentration, sleep difficulties, sexual dysfunction, social avoidance, irritability, and drug or alcohol abuse.[200] The chronic stress-related conditions and disorders resulting from severe weather or other climate change-related events may lead to additional negative health effects. Studies have shown a negative relationship between stress and blood glucose levels, including influence on glycemic control among patients with type 2 diabetes.[201] Evidence has also shown that human response to repeated episodes of acute psychological stress or to chronic psychological stress may result in cardiovascular disease.[202] Although a direct cause and effect relationship has not yet been proven, some research has indicated a link between various psychological factors and an increased risk of developing

191 Kessler, RC, et al., Arch Gen Psychiatry, 2005. 62(6): p. 617-27.
192 Ibid.
193 Fritze, JG, et al., Int J Ment Health Syst, 2008. 2(1): p. 13.
194 Ibid.
195 Ibid.
196 Ibid.

197 Martin-Latry, K, et al., Eur Psychiatry, 2007. 22(6): p. 335-8.
198 Tapsell, SM, et al., Philos Transact A Math Phys Eng Sci, 2002. 360(1796): p. 1511-25.
199 Ebi, K, et al. In Analyses of the effects of global change on human health and welfare and human systems. A Report by the U.S. Climate Change Science Program and the Subcommittee on Global Change Research, J Gamble, et al., Editors. 2008, USEPA: Washington, D. C.
200 Silove, D, et al., J Postgrad Med, 2006. 52(2): p. 121-5, Weisler, RH, et al. JAMA, 2006. 296(5): p. 585-8.
201 Surwit, RS, et al., Diabetes Care, 2002. 25(1): p. 30-4.
202 Black, PH, et al., J Psychosom Res, 2002. 52(1): p. 1-23.

some forms of cancer, as well as the progression of cancer in those already presenting with the disease.[203]

Climate change has the potential to create sustained natural and humanitarian disasters beyond the scale of those we are experiencing today, which may exceed the capacity of our public health systems to cope with societal demands.[204] In the United States, this was demonstrated in 2005 by the devastating impact of Hurricane Katrina. Globally, climate change will continue to act as a threat to natural resources and ecosystem services that are already stressed, which may force the migration of large communities and create conditions leading to hostile political environments, conflict, and war.[205] The resources required to meet the psychological needs of those affected by extreme weather events, environmental conflicts, or other effects of climate change may be limited immediately following such an event,[206] or as people migrate in search of more stable natural environments.

Research on mental health service delivery following disaster events has only recently become a higher profile topic of scientific interest. Though some mental health diseases and stress-related disorders have been incorporated into the collection of health impacts of extreme weather and temperature events, numerous research gaps remain. More work is necessary to understand the effects of climate change and extreme weather events on mental health status, to determine how to mitigate these effects, and to overcome the barriers to utilization and delivery of mental health services following extreme weather events.

Impacts on Risks

The number of people killed by climatic, hydrological, and meteorological disasters in 2008 was the highest of the last decade, with 147,722 deaths reported worldwide.[207] In the United States, Hurricanes Katrina and Rita, which hit the Gulf Coast in 2005, were two of the most damaging hurricanes recorded in U.S. history, impacting more than 90,000 square miles and directly affecting more than 1.5 million people, including forcing 800,000 citizens to be relocated from their homes.[208] Scientific evidence supports that global warming will be accompanied by changes in the intensity, duration, and geographical extent of weather and climate extreme events; therefore, the threat to human health and well being from

events such as hurricanes, wildfires, flooding, and tornadoes is likely to continue, and perhaps worsen.[209]

It is also highly likely that the long-term effects of climate change will displace significant numbers of people, many of whom are already vulnerable members of society. Extreme weather events, sea-level rise, destruction of local economies, resource scarcity, and associated conflict due to climate change are predicted to displace millions of people worldwide over the coming century.[210] The most commonly cited figure of projected population displacement from climate change is 200 million people worldwide by 2050.[211] Those with lower socio-economic standing are more likely to choose to relocate permanently following a devastating event, often due to limited resources to rebuild property and restore livelihood.[212] In addition, people will continue to experience place-based distress caused by the effects of climate change due to involuntary migration or the loss of connection to one's home environment, a phenomenon called "Solastalgia."[213]

The mental health impacts of environmentally displaced populations in conflict stricken areas have been well documented;[214] however, additional research is needed to better understand mental health impacts on such people as they relate to climate change and climate change-related migration. While there wil likely be some displacement of populations in the United States caused by the effects of climate change, this issue is anticipated to have far greater consequences on a global scale. The results of climate science research on sea-level rise, extreme events such as flooding and droughts, the impacts of climate change on natural resources, and other impacts caused by climate variability and change must be connected to social science research. This link to social sciences, including behavioral science research, will help to build an understanding of when, how, and where population shifts may occur, thereby increasing the likelihood that necessary mental health services and support can be made available where and when they are needed most.

203 Antoni, MH, et al., Nat Rev Cancer, 2006. 6(3): p. 240-8.
204 The CNA Corporation, 2007. p. 68.
205 Kessler, RC, et al., Arch Gen Psychiatry, 2005. 62(6): p. 617-27.
206 Tapsell, SM, et al., Philos Transact A Math Phys Eng Sci, 2002. 360(1796): p. 1511-25.
207 International Federation of Red Cross and Red Crescent Societies, World Disaster Report 2009, In World Disaster Report, L. Knight, Editor. 2009, International Federation of Red Cross and Red Crescent Societies: Geneva. p. 210.
208 Department of Homeland Security. The First Year After Hurricane Katrina: What the Federal Government Did., 2009 [cited 2009 July 22]; Available from: www.dhs.gov/xfoia/archives/gc_1157649340100.shtm.

209 CCSP. Weather and Climate Extremes in a Changing Climate. Regions of Focus: North America, Hawaii, Caribbean, and U.S. Pacific Islands. A Report by the U.S. Climate Change Science Program and the Subcommittee on Global Change Research., T. Karl, et al., Editors. 2008, Department of Commerce, NOAA's National Climatic Data Center: Washington, DC, USA. p. 164.
210 Fritze, JG, et al., Int J Ment Health Syst, 2008. 2(1): p. 13.
211 Myers, N, Philos Trans R Soc Lond B Biol Sci, 2002. 357(1420): p. 609-13.
212 Hunter, LM, Population and Environment, 2005. 26(4): p. 273-302.
213 Albrecht, G, et al., Australasian Psychiatry, 2007. 15: p. 595-598.
214 Crowley, C, J Am Acad Nurse Pract, 2009. 21(6): p. 322-31; Mills, E, et al., Med Confl Surviv, 2008. 24(1): p. 5-15; Naeem, F, et al., J Ayub Med Coll Abbottabad, 2005. 17(2): p. 23-5; Hollifield, M, et al., Jama, 2002. 288(5): p. 611-21.

Mitigation and Adaptation

There is a need to fully understand what gaps currently exist in mental health infrastructure, resources, and services; how these gaps may be exacerbated due to climate change; and the resulting impacts on mental health status, both in the United States and worldwide. This information can then be incorporated into mitigation and adaptation strategies. The information can also be used to ensure adequate resources are allocated to enable services to prepare for and deal with the impending challenges associated with climate change including both extreme and chronic weather events and sea-level rise. In addition, much work needs to be done to help individuals better self-identify their mental health needs and to increase their awareness of the existence of mental health services in their communities. Work also needs to be done to eradicate the stigma associated with the need for mental health care so that individuals will seek out mental health services following extreme weather or other climate-related events.

While some climate change adaptation measures may prevent the need for displacement and migration of communities, socioeconomically disadvantaged communities both within the United States and globally may not be able to effectively implement such adaptation measures. The effect may be social instability of the surrounding community, which will create additional stress and exacerbate the threat to overall mental health and well being.

Research Needs

Immediate research needs on the mental health implications of climate change[215] include:

- understanding of how psychological stress acts synergistically with other forms of environmental exposures to cause adverse mental health effects

- understanding the critical social and economic determinants for mental health and overall community well-being that might be altered by climate change

- identifying and incorporating key mental health outcomes in health impact assessments, both for U.S. populations and worldwide, under a range of climate change scenarios

- developing and implementing monitoring networks to help track the migration of environmentally displaced populations to assist with the provision of mental health care and services

- improving methods of identifying vulnerable mental health populations, and understanding the implications for these populations at the local and regional level

- identifying the most beneficial means of encouraging utilization of mental health services and delivering such services following extreme weather or other climate change events

- developing mental health promotion and communication programs related to proposed climate change mitigation and adaptation strategies

---

215 Fritze, JG, et al., Int J Ment Health Syst, 2008. 2(1): p. 13.

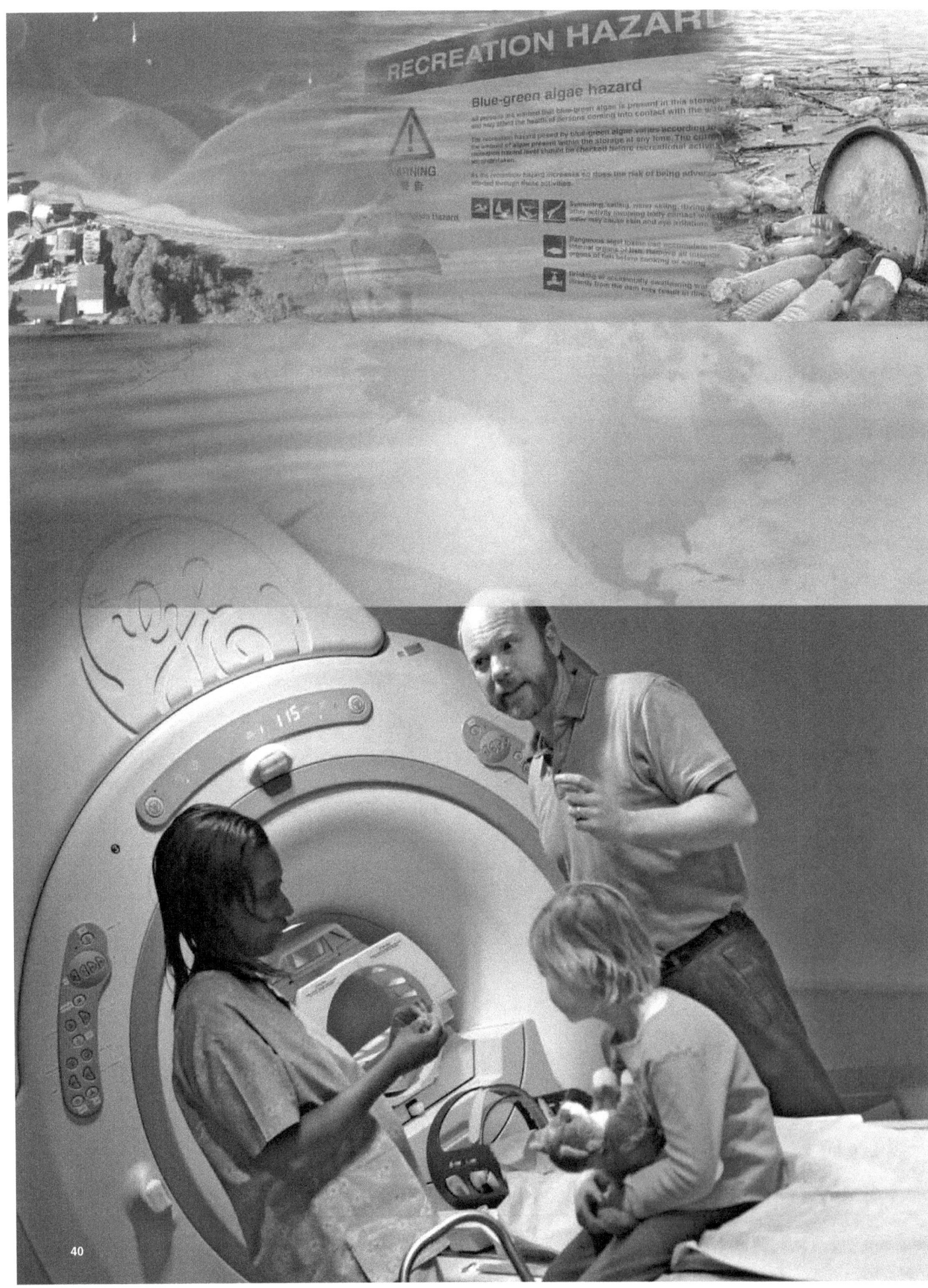

Neurological Diseases and Disorders

The United States has seen an increasing trend in the prevalence of neurological diseases and deficits.[216] Onset of diseases such as Alzheimer Disease (AD) and Parkinson Disease (PD) is occurring at earlier ages across the population. Environmental factors are suspected of playing a large role in both the onset and severity of these conditions, although there is a gap in our understanding of this role, especially in relation to genetics, aging, and other factors.[217] While some of these changes in neurological health likely are due to the aging of a large portion of the population, learning disabilities that affect children also are on the rise, and there are indicators that environmental factors may be involved including changes in climate that may exacerbate factors affecting the rates and severity of neurological conditions.[218,219] Neurological conditions generally carry high costs in terms of quality of life for both the sufferer and the caregiver and increased healthcare stresses on the economy and the workforce. The combination of these factors could affect a sizable portion of the U.S. population, and have significant impacts on productivity.

Factors affected by climate with particular implications for neurological functioning include malnutrition;[220] exposure to hazardous chemicals, biotoxins, and metals in air, food, and water;[221] and changes in pest management.[222] Understanding the role of climate in the incidence and progression of neurological conditions and how to prevent them is a critical need for public health and health care in the United States. Studies such as the National Children's Study[223] are an excellent opportunity to improve our understanding in this area.

Impacts on Risk

Numerous recent reports have described observed and anticipated detrimental effects of climate change on ocean health, resulting in increased risks to neurological health from ingestion of or

RESEARCH HIGHLIGHT

Harmful algal blooms (HABs) are increasing worldwide and global climate change is thought to play a significant role. Many HAB-related biotoxins cause significant neurotoxic effects in both animals and humans including permanent neurological impairment. The algae *Pseudonitzschia* spp. produce domoic acid, a potent neurotoxin that causes amnesiac shellfish poisoning in people. Blooms of this algae have been increasing off the California coast resulting in significant illness and death in marine animals. A decade of monitoring of health of California sea lions, a sentinel species for human health effects, indicates changes in the neurologic symptomatology and epidemiology of domoic acid toxicosis. Three separate clinical syndromes are now present in exposed animals: acute domoic acid toxicosis with seizure, permanent hippocampal atrophy, and death; a second novel neurological syndrome characterized by epilepsy associated with the chronic consequences of sub-lethal exposure to domoic acid; and a third syndrome associated with *in utero* exposures resulting in premature parturition, neonatal death, and significant neurotoxicity in the developing fetus resulting in seizure activity as the animal grows, as well as long-lasting impacts on memory and learning.[1] These observations indicate significant potential implications for human health effects, although their exact nature is not known and needs further study.

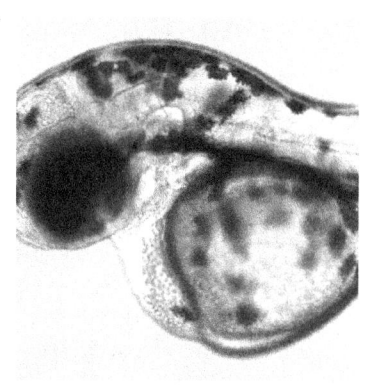

216 Steenland, K, et al., Alzheimer Dis Assoc Disord, 2009. 23(2): p. 165-70.
217 Bronstein, J, et al., Environmental Health Perspectives, 2009. 117(1): p. 117-121, Hendrie, HC, et al., Canadian Journal of Psychiatry-Revue Canadienne De Psychiatrie, 2004. 49(2): p. 92-99, Mayeux, R, Annals of Neurology, 2004. 55(2): p. 156-158.
218 Bronstein, J, et al., Environmental Health Perspectives, 2009. 117(1): p. 117-121, Mayeux, R, Annals of Neurology, 2004. 55(2): p. 156-158, Jones, L, et al., Lancet, 2009. 374(9690): p. 654-61.
219 Altevogt, BM, et al., Pediatrics, 2008. 121(6): p. 1225-1229.
220 Kar, BR, et al., Behav Brain Funct, 2008. 4: p. 31.
221 Kozma, C, Am J Med Genet A, 2005. 132(4): p. 441-4, Papanikolaou, NC, et al., Med Sci Monit, 2005. 11(10): p. RA329-36.
222 Handal, AJ, et al., Epidemiology, 2007. 18(3): p. 312-20.
223 Landrigan, PJ, et al., Pediatrics, 2006. 118(5): p. 2173-86.

1 Goldstein, T, et al., Proceedings of the Royal Society B-Biological Sciences, 2008. 275(1632): p. 267-276. Ramsdell, JS and TS Zabka, Marine drugs, 2008. 6(2): p. 262-90.

exposure to neurotoxins in seafood and fresh and marine waters.[224] Neurotoxins produced by harmful algal blooms and other marine microorganisms can cause serious illness and death in humans. Under the correct conditions, harmful algal blooms produce potent neurotoxins that are often taken up and bioaccumulated in filter-feeding molluscan shellfish including oysters, clams, and mussels, as well as by certain marine and freshwater fish.[225] The most frequent human exposures are via consumption of seafood containing algal toxins, although some toxins may be present in freshwater sources of drinking water, and others may be aerosolized by surf breaking on beaches and then transported by winds to where they can cause respiratory distress in susceptible individuals who breathe them.[226] Because cooking or other means of food preparation do not kill seafood biotoxins, it is essential to identify contaminated seafood before it reaches consumers. Health effects including amnesia, diarrhea, numbness, liver damage, skin and eye irritation, respiratory paralysis, and PD- and AD-like symptoms may be severe, chronic, and even lead to death.[227] It has recently been reported that even a single low-level exposure to algal toxins can result in physiological changes indicative of neurodegeneration.[228] Work done on biotoxin-related neurologic disease in marine mammals indicates that domoic acid exposure can cause acute neurologic symptoms by crossing the placenta and accumulating in the amniotic fluid where it can impact neural development in the fetus, alter postnatal development, and lead to chronic illnesses such as epilepsy.[229,230,231] Climate change may alter the geographic range in which harmful algal bloom toxins appear, the frequency of toxin production, and the actual delivery of toxins (both increasing and decreasing in some cases) due to extreme weather.[232] Harmful algal blooms are increasing in frequency, intensity, and duration globally, partially as a result of climate change, although this link is poorly understood.[233] Nonetheless, it is clear that changes in precipitation and ocean temperatures, coupled with increased nutrient loading, may lead to earlier seasonal occurrence, as well as longer lasting and possibly more toxic harmful algal blooms.[234]

Emerging research suggests that exposure to a number of agents whose environmental presence may increase with climate change may have effects on neurological development and functioning. For example, exposure to pesticides and herbicides during specific developmental windows, in combination with other exposures later in life, could increase the risk of PD and other neurological diseases.[235] Exposure to heavy metals is known to exacerbate neurological deficits and learning disabilities in children,[236] and is suspected of being associated with both onset and exacerbation of AD[237] and PD. Evidence suggests that early-life occurrence of inflammation in the brain, as a consequence of either brain injury or exposure to infectious agents, also may play a role in the pathogenesis of PD.[238] In addition to conditions such as PD and AD, post-traumatic stress disorder (PTSD) is likely to have profound effects on the neurological functioning of populations exposed to the stress of extreme weather events, and the resulting dislocation and deprivation that may result from climate change.[239]

Mitigation and Adaptation

Mitigation to climate change may reduce our reliance on fossil fuels. This reduction in fossil fuel use will reduce the release of a number of neurotoxicants including arsenic, mercury, and other metals into the environment.[240] Simple actions that reduce the amount of energy needed, such as expanded use of compact fluorescent light bulbs, will reduce the amount of toxic metals emitted into the air by coal-fired power plants. However, additional mercury releases into the environment might occur due to breakage of these fluorescent bulbs or improper disposal, resulting in human exposures and potential neurological effects.[241] In more complicated mitigation strategies such as the expansion of the use of electric vehicles, heavy metals used in the batteries for such vehicles may present manufacturing and disposal challenges that will be of particular significance to the risk of neurological deficits.[242]

Adaptation efforts such as the increased use of pesticides to improve crop yield in areas with reduced farming capabilities may result in runoff of potentially neurotoxic pesticides into reservoirs and coasts used to capture water for human use, thereby increasing

224 National Research Council (U.S.). Committee on Ecological Impacts of Climate Change. 2008, Washington, D.C.: National Academies Press. xii, 57 p.; Sandifer, P., et al., Interagency oceans and human health research implementation plan: a prescription for the future. 2007, Interagency Working Group on Harmful Algal Blooms, Hypoxia and Human Health of the Joint Subcommittee on Ocean Science and Technology: Washington, DC, USA.

225 Wang, DZ, Marine Drugs, 2008. 6(2): p. 349–71.

226 Kirkpatrick, B, et al., Sci Total Environ, 2008. 402(1): p. 1–8.

227 Wang, DZ, Marine Drugs, 2008. 6(2): p. 349–71.

228 Lefebvre, KA, et al., Toxicol Sci, 2009. 107(1): p. 65–77.

229 Ramsdell, JS, et al., Marine Drugs, 2008. 6(2): p. 262–90.

230 Brodie, EC, et al., Marine Mammal Science, 2006. 22(3): p. 700–707.

231 Maucher, JM, et al., Environmental Health Perspectives, 2007. 115(12): p. 1743–1746.

232 Moore, SK, et al., Environmental Health: A Global Access Science Source, 2008. 7(SUPPL. 2); Sandifer, P, et al., Interagency oceans and human health research implementation plan: a prescription for the future. 2007, Interagency Working Group on Harmful Algal Blooms, Hypoxia and Human Health of the Joint Subcommittee on Ocean Science and Technology: Washington, DC, USA.

233 Moore, SK, et al., Environmental Health: A Global Access Science Source, 2008. 7(SUPPL. 2).

234 Paerl, HW, et al., Science, 2008. 320(5872): p. 57–8.

235 Costello, S, et al., Am J Epidemiol, 2009. 169(8): p. 919–26.

236 Kozma, C, Am J Med Genet A, 2005. 132(4): p. 441–4.

237 Kotermanski, SE, et al., J Neurosci, 2009. 29(9): p. 2774–9, Lovell, MA, J Alzheimers Dis, 2009. 16(3): p. 471–83, Mendes, CT, et al., Eur Arch Psychiatry Clin Neurosci, 2009. 259(1): p. 16–22, Quinn, JF, et al., Expert Rev Neurother, 2009. 9(5): p. 631–7.

238 Miller, DB, et al., Metabolism, 2008. 57 Suppl 2: p. S44–9.

239 Naeem, F, et al., J Ayub Med Coll Abbottabad, 2005. 17(2): p. 23–5.

240 Gustin, MS, et al., J Air Waste Manag Assoc, 2004. 54(3): p. 320–30. Narukawa, T, et al., J Environ Monit, 2005. 7(12): p. 1342–8, Ito, S, et al., Sci Total Environ, 2006. 368(1): p. 397–402.

241 Noyes, PD, et al., Environment International, 2009. 35(6): p. 971–986.

242 Bronstein, J, et al., Environmental Health Perspectives, 2009. 117(1): p. 117–121.

human exposures.[243] Alternately, recent research has shown multiple benefits on mental and neurological functioning as a result of increased exposure to natural and green space settings, particularly in urban areas.[244] Adaptation strategies that encourage and allow walkable cities and exercise, increases in green space and urban forestry, and improved green building methods that reduce the potential for exposure to chemicals such as arsenic and lead that leach from building materials could all contribute to reductions in neurological deficits. Numerous other mitigation and adaptation strategies may have both positive and negative health effects, most of which are poorly recognized or understood. Thus, any proposed mitigation and adaptation strategies will need to be carefully evaluated for both benefits and potential neurological effects.

Research Needs

More research is needed regarding the link between environmental exposures, the onset and severity of neurological diseases and disorders, and the relationship to climate change. Research needs include:

- identifying the factors that initiate harmful algal blooms and bacterial proliferations, focusing on the effects of temperature changes, shifts in rainfall patterns, and other climate-associated factors on their distribution, occurrence, and severity

- improving understanding of the mechanisms and pathways of acute and chronic exposures to harmful algal biotoxins and their impacts on fetal, postnatal, and adult development

- utilizing marine animal models to better understand the mechanisms and outcomes of exposure to harmful algal biotoxins individually and in conjunction with chemical exposures

- developing and validating strategies to inhibit the formation and severity of harmful algal blooms

- expanding research on the toxicity of chemicals known or suspected to cause neurological disorders, particularly pesticides, and on understanding how climate change may affect human exposure to such chemicals

- improving our understanding of the impact of increased heavy precipitation, ice melts, and flooding events on the risk of toxic contamination of the environment from storage-related issues or runoff, focusing on the likelihood of the event, the geographical areas and populations likely to be impacted, and the health outcomes that could result

- examining the neurological health benefits and costs of new climate change mitigation technologies, including research on the toxicity of new metals and metal compounds, including nanotechnologies, being used to improve battery performance for electric vehicles

243 Noyes, PD, et al., Environment International, 2009. 35(6): p. 971-986.
244 Frumkin, H, et al. 2004. Washington, DC: Island Press. xxi, 338 p.

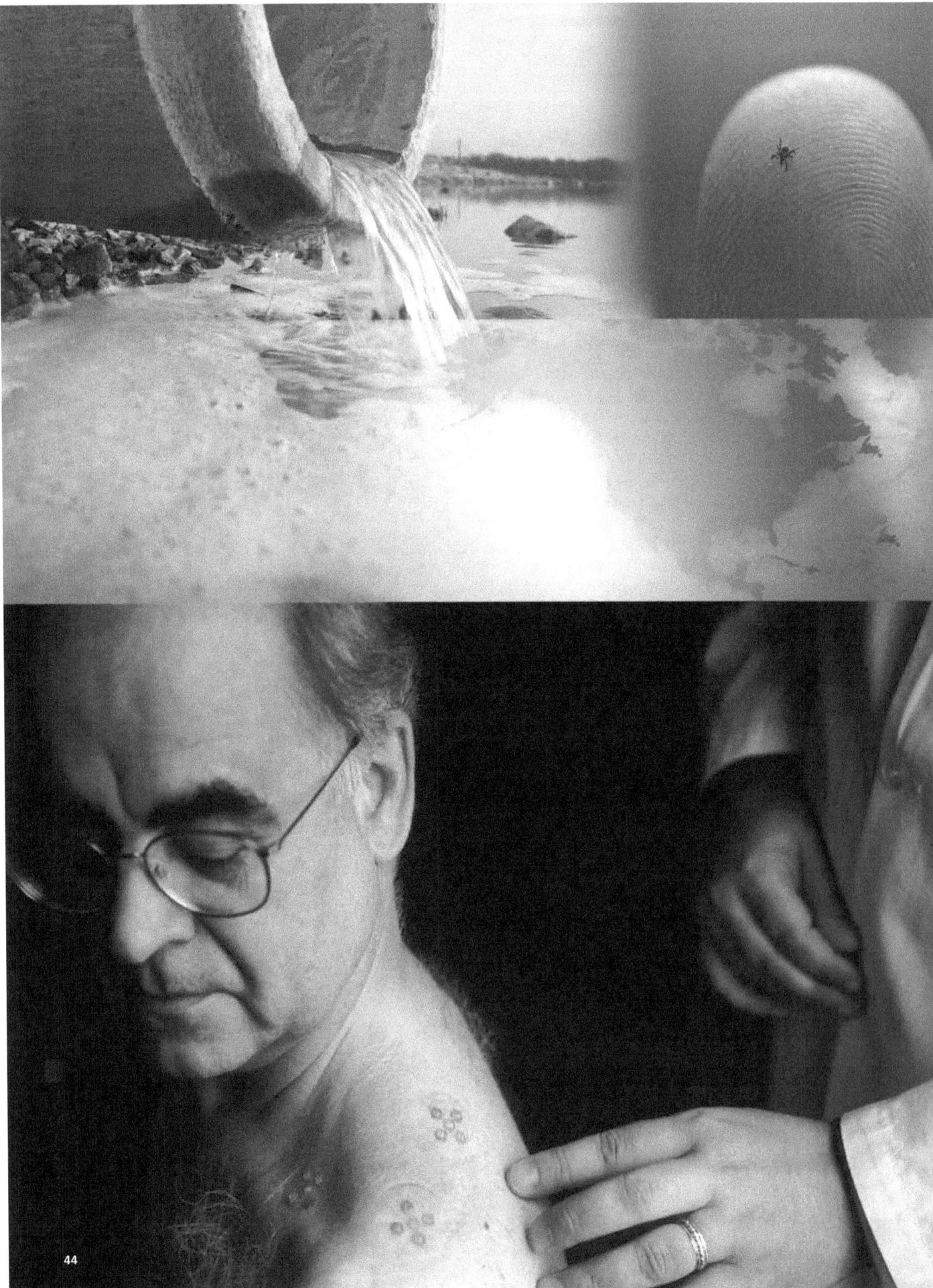

Vectorborne and Zoonotic Disease

Vectorborne and zoonotic diseases (VBZD) are infectious diseases whose transmission cycles involve animal hosts or vectors. Vectorborne diseases are those in which organisms, typically blood-feeding arthropods (insects, ticks, or mites) carry the pathogen from one host to another, generally with amplification (increased virulence) in the vector (for example, malaria). Zoonoses are diseases that can be transmitted from animals to humans by either contact with animals or by vectors that can carry zoonotic pathogens from animals to humans (for example, avian flu). Both domestic animals and wildlife, including marine mammals, fish, sea turtles, and seabirds may play roles in VBZD transmission by serving as zoonotic reservoirs for human pathogens or as means of interspecies transmission of pathogens. The epidemiology of VBZD in the United States has changed significantly over the past century, and many diseases that previously caused significant illness and death, including malaria,[245] dengue,[246] yellow fever,[247] and murine typhus,[248] are now rarely seen in this country. This dramatic change is a result of intentional programs to control vectors, vaccinate against disease, and detect and treat cases, with additional benefits from improvements in sanitation, development, and environmental modification. Examples of vectorborne diseases currently prevalent in the United States include Lyme disease[249] and ehrlichiosis, bacterial diseases that are transmitted primarily by ticks. Other important zoonoses in the United States, some of which are also vectorborne, include rabies,[250] Q fever,[251] anthrax, pathogenic *E. coli*, tularemia, hantavirus pulmonary syndrome,[252] and plague. Although VBZD currently are not a leading cause of morbidity or mortality in the United States, there is cause for some urgency on this issue. Our population is directly susceptible to the VBZD that circulate in warmer climates, and vulnerable as a result of global trade and travel. Our ability to respond to such threats on both a national and international level is currently limited.

Many vectorborne diseases that have been virtually eliminated from the industrialized world are still prevalent in developing countries. Globally, VBZD cause significant morbidity and mortality. For

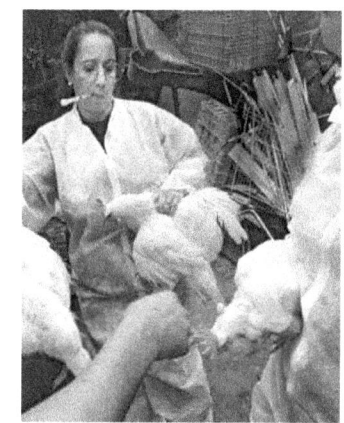

RESEARCH HIGHLIGHT

Climate is one of several factors that influence the distribution of vectorborne and zoonotic diseases (VBZD) such as Lyme disease, Hantavirus, West Nile virus, and malaria. There is substantial concern that climate change will make certain environments more suitable for some VBZD, worsening their already significant global burden and potentially reintroducing some diseases into geographic areas where they had been previously eradicated. Recent public health experience with the outbreak and establishment of West Nile virus in the United States reveals the complexity of such epidemics, and the lack of preparedness required by public health officials to contain a national VBZD threat. Though unlikely, West Nile virus might have been contained when it emerged in New York City in 1999; however, delays of only a few weeks in recognizing the outbreak in birds and identifying the virus, combined with the absence of a robust mosquito abatement capability, allowed West Nile virus to spread quickly to surrounding areas. Relying on expertise from the mosquito abatement community, aerial spraying was applied fairly rapidly to combat mosquitoes in infected areas, but these efforts were not adequate to decrease populations of mosquitoes in time. From New York, the virus traveled across the entire United States, and by 2003, it had thoroughly established itself in the avian population. To date, individual mosquito abatement districts have been able to significantly protect their populations due to increased national funding combined with decades of experience in their local areas. However, underserved regions did not get significant protection despite efforts to identify them.

Resurgence of vectorborne disease as a result of climate change is also a major concern. Despite energetic interventions, the availability of drugs

245 Faust, E. In Malariology: a comprehensive survey of all aspects of this group of diseases from a global standpoint, MF Boyd, Editor. 1949, Saunders: Philadelphia,. p. 2 v. (xxl, 1643 p.).
246 Adler, P, et al., American Entomologist, 2003. 49: p. 216-229.
247 Petri, WA, Jr., Am J Trop Med Hyg, 2004. 71(1): p. 2-16.
248 White, PC, Jr., Mil Med, 1965. 130: p. 386-8.
249 Bacon, RM, et al., MMWR Surveill Summ, 2008. 57(10): p. 1-9.
250 Blanton, JD, et al., J Am Vet Med Assoc, 2008. 233(6): p. 884-97.
251 McQuiston, JH, et al., Am J Trop Med Hyg, 2006. 75(1): p. 36-40.
252 Douglass, RJ, et al., Vector Borne Zoonotic Dis, 2005. 5(2): p. 189-92.

example, in 2006 there were 247 million cases of malaria and 881,000 malaria-related deaths worldwide.[253] The World Health Organization estimates that malaria is responsible for 2.9% of the world's total disability-adjusted life years (DALYs).[254] In the long term, climate change's potential to cause social upheaval and population displacement may provide opportunities for resurgence of certain VBZD in the United States, which has already seen some redistribution of vector species.[255] Disruption of economies, transportation routes, agriculture, and environmental services could result in large-scale population movements within and between countries, as well as a general decrease in what are now considered minimum standards of living.[256] A severe degradation of rural and urban climate and sanitation conditions could bring malaria, epidemic typhus, plague, and yellow fever to their former prominence.

Valid projections on likely impacts of climate change on VBZD are lacking, and a scientific consensus has yet to emerge. Even though we now have the technical knowledge to treat or vaccinate against many VBZD, in the absence of these technologies, some experts believe that population-level mortality from certain disease outbreaks could reach as high as 20–50%.[257] Ultimately, projections must be specific to location, altitude, ecosystem, and host or vector. Health impacts from changing distributions of VBZD are likely to unfold over the next several decades, and prevention and control activities must be developed and honed prior to significant vector range expansion in order to be most effective.

Emerging zoonotic disease outbreaks are increasing, with the majority of recent major human infectious disease outbreaks worldwide, as well as significant emerging diseases such as SARS, Nipah virus, and HIV/AIDS, originating in animals.[258] A recent report noted that the United States remains the world's largest importer of wildlife, both legal and illegal; these animals represent a potential source of zoonotic pathogen introduction into U.S. communities.[259] Interactions of wildlife with domestic animals and with people will likely increase in the United States due to changes to ecosystems and disease transmission resulting from both climate change and from adaptation and response strategies.

Impacts on Risks

VBZD ecology is complex, and weather and climate are among several factors that influence transmission cycles and human disease incidence.[260] Impacts in certain ecosystems are better understood; however, for others such as marine ecosystems, their role in VBZD has not been well characterized.[261] Changes in temperature and precipitation patterns affect VBZD directly through pathogen-host-vector interactions, and indirectly through ecosystem changes (humidity, soil moisture, water temperature, salinity, acidity) and species composition. Social and cultural behaviors also affect disease transmission. Many VBZD exhibit some degree of climate sensitivity, and ecological shifts associated with climate variability and long-term climate change are expected to impact the distribution and incidence of many of these diseases.[262] For instance, the range of Lyme disease is expected to expand northward as the range of the deer tick that transmits it expands.[263] In another example, the frequency of hantavirus pulmonary syndrome outbreaks, caused by human exposure to the virus in deer mice urine or feces, may change with increasingly variable rainfall in the desert Southwest, which affects the populations of deer mice and other rodents through changes in production of the pine nuts on which they feed.[264]

Similarly, certain VBZD may decrease in particular regions as habitats become less suitable for host or vector populations and for sustained disease transmission. Coastal and marine ecosystems will be particularly impacted by increasing temperatures, changes in precipitation patterns, sea-level rise, altered salinity, ocean acidification, and more frequent and intense extreme weather events. These changes will directly and indirectly affect ocean and coastal ecosystems by influencing community structure, biodiversity, and the growth, survival, persistence, distribution, transmission, and severity of disease-causing organisms, vectors, and reservoirs.[265] Also of concern for both terrestrial and aquatic/marine ecosystems is the loss of biodiversity (which underlies ecosystem services) that further exacerbates the impacts of climate change on vectors or animal reservoir populations. Such alterations in ecosystem functions may alter the emergence of VBZD in populations within the United States. With the loss of predators, insect vectors may increase, making necessary either chemical or mechanical controls.

253 WHO. Global Malaria Programme. 2008, Geneva: World Health Organization. xx, 190 p.

254 WHO. 2002, Geneva: World Health Organization. xx, 190 p.

255 Carroll, JF, Proc. of the Entomological Society of Washington, 2007. 109(1): p. 253-256.

256 Costello, A, et al., The Lancet, 2009. 373(9676): p. 1693-1733.

257 Orenstein, WA, et al., Health Aff (Millwood), 2005. 24(3): p. 599-610.

258 Institute of Medicine (U.S.). Committee on Achieving Sustainable Global Capacity for Surveillance and Response to Emerging Diseases of Zoonotic Origin., et al. 2009, Washington, DC: National Academies Press. xxv, 312 p.

259 Pavlin, BI, et al., Emerg Infect Dis, 2009. 15(11): p. 1721-6.

260 Boxall, ABA, et al., Environmental Health Perspectives, 2009. 117(4): p. 508-514.

261 Constantin de Magny, G, et al., Trans Am Clin Climatol Assoc, 2009. 120: p. 119-28.

262 Gage, KL, et al., Am J Prev Med, 2008. 35(5): p. 436-50.

263 Estrada-Peña, A, Environ Health Perspect, 2002. 110(7): p. 635-40.

264 Douglass, RJ, et al., Vector Borne Zoonotic Dis, 2005. 5(2): p. 189-92, Costello, A, et al., The Lancet, 2009. 373(9676): p. 1693-1733, Ebi, KL, et al., Environmental Health Perspectives, 2006. 114(9): p. 1318-1324.

265 Niemi, G, et al., Environmental Health Perspectives, 2004. 112(9): p. 979-986.

Projecting VBZD incidence is difficult given the complexity of VBZD transmission cycles, the variability of regional and local impacts of climate change, and the limited information currently available regarding the ecology of many VBZD. For instance, while malaria transmission increases with temperature and humidity, the decrease in disease incidence seen with prolonged drought may negate these effects. Human rural and urban development efforts, such as the creation of clean water sources for animal husbandry or swamp clearance to increase availability of land for human settlement, also have significant impacts on transmission dynamics that can offset climate impacts.

The incidence of VBZD in the United States will likely increase under anticipated climate change scenarios, for several reasons. The distribution of vectors currently restricted to warmer climates will expand into the United States. For example, the habitats of two potent mosquito vectors of malaria, *Anopheles albimanus* and *Anopheles pseudopunctipennis*, currently range as far north as northern Mexico, and would presumably expand northwards across the U.S.–Mexico border.[266] The extrinsic incubation period of pathogens in invertebrate vectors is highly dependent on ambient temperature. Since the lifespan of vector species is relatively constant, changes in the incubation period due to precipitation and temperature significantly alter the likelihood of transmission.[267] Also, large disruption and subsequent movement of human populations create conditions for wider distribution of pathogens and greater exposure to vector species.[268] And, climate change is already affecting the biodiversity of marine and terrestrial ecosystems, which in turn will alter the dynamics of predator–prey relationships, as well as vector and reservoir pathogen populations. This may alter the types and quality of subsistence animal foods, and present dependent communities with new pathogen risks.[269] The time scale of this threat will be continuous unless mitigating measures are taken. Economic and regulatory restrictions continue to slow the development and use of new modes of action against vectors.

RESEARCH HIGHLIGHT continued

for treatment, and vector control strategies supported by strong scientific understanding, malaria continues to be a severe problem in Africa and a persistent one in Asia and Latin America. Malaria could present a threatened return to its former importance in more temperate climates.[1] Korea provides a recent case study with respect to the more chronic, less fatal species of the parasite, *Plasmodium vivax*.[2] Malaria became a severe problem on the Korean peninsula during and following the Korean War in 1950–1953. A combination of case detection, treatment, and vector control reduced the number of cases and finally eliminated the parasite from South Korea by 1988.[3] The disease reemerged in 1993 and quickly became a problem in the military population by 1996, with cases of temperate-adapted parasites exported to the United States.[4] Subsequent studies of the vector mosquitoes revealed that a complex of multiple species, including a powerful vector, *Anopheles anthropophagus* that is prevalent in China, is responsible for the reemergence. This reemergence may have been exacerbated by increases in severe rainfall events and temperature, but this has not yet been definitively established.[5]

The story is different in sub-Saharan Africa, where malaria is responsible for a large proportion of the infant and childhood mortality.[6] Researchers have examined whether the wider distribution of malaria in highland regions is associated with climate change, and have performed quantitative predictions of the effects of various climate change scenarios on distribution of the disease.[7] Climate change induced increases in temperature may have several effects: increase the altitude at which malaria transmission is possible, intensify transmission at lower altitudes, and generally make greater demands on the efficacy of vector control efforts.

1 Faust, E. in Malariology; a comprehensive survey of all aspects of this group of diseases from a global standpoint, MF Boyd, Editor. 1949, Saunders: Philadelphia., p. 2 v. (xxi, 1643 p.).
2 Ree, HI, Korean J Parasitol, 2000. 38(3): p. 119-38.
3 Paik, YH, et al., Jpn J Exp Med, 1988. 58(2): p. 55-66.
4 Feighner, BH, et al., Emerg Infect Dis, 1998. 4(2): p. 295-7.
5 Foley, DH, et al., J Med Entomol, 2009. 46(3): p. 680-92.
6 WHO, Global Malaria Programme. 2008, Geneva: World Health Organization. xx, 190 p.
7 Ebi, KL, et al., Climatic Change, 2005. 73(3): p. 375-393, Thomson, MC, et al., Trends in Parasitology, 2001. 17(9): p. 438-445, Zhou, G, et al., Trends Parasitol, 2005. 21(2): p. 54-6.

266 Rogers, DJ, et al., Science, 2000. 289(5485): p. 1763-6.
267 Strickman, D, et al., American Journal of Tropical Medicine and Hygiene, 2003. 68(2): p. 209-217.
268 Scoville, A. in Rickettsial diseases of man; a symposium, FR Moulton, Editor. 1948, American Association for the Advancement of Science.: Washington, D.C., p. 247 p.
269 Niemi, G, et al., Environmental Health Perspectives, 2004. 112(9): p. 979-986, Jentsch, A, et al., Comptes Rendus Geoscience, 2008. 340(9-10): p. 621-628.

Mitigation and Adaptation

Climate change mitigation includes activities to reduce greenhouse gas emissions such as decreased reliance on fossil fuels for energy generation and transport and changes in land use such as reducing deforestation and conversion of forested land to cropland. Strategies focused on alternative energy sources with lower greenhouse gas emission profiles, such as nuclear power, may influence local ecologies by increasing water demands, temperature, and currents.[270,271] This, in turn, might alter the life cycles of certain disease vectors and animals that are part of VBZD transmission cycles. Increased reliance on hydroelectric power, which typically requires construction of dams, also may change local VBZD ecologies and alter transmission cycles. Mitigation activities focused on land use changes, particularly preservation of forests and wetlands, are likely to impact VBZD ecology and transmission cycles as well.[270] For example, changes to wetlands may affect mosquito burden in certain areas by altering breeding area size and potentially altering the incidence of malaria, dengue, or other mosquito-borne diseases.[271] Because the margins of disturbed ecosystems can be associated with outbreaks of zoonotic infections such as Ebola and Marburg viruses,[272] ecosystem preservation may also reduce the incidence of these VBZD. The net impact, either beneficial or detrimental, of these mitigations strategies on human health is difficult to determine, and more research is needed to elucidate these effects.

Climate change adaptation strategies include activities that provide early warning and reduce exposure to environmental hazards associated with climate change, and limit susceptibility in exposed populations. Some adaptation activities may impact VBZD or alter the potential for human exposure. For example, encouraging air conditioning use as an adaptation strategy against extreme heat may provide a co-benefit of reduced exposure to VBZD. The use of central air conditioning has been shown to be a protective factor against dengue infection in studies comparing dengue incidence on opposite sides of the U.S.-Mexico border.[273] Negative impacts of adaptation are also possible. For example, capture and storage of water runoff to adapt to increasingly sporadic rainfall might provide more suitable breeding habitat for mosquitoes, thereby increasing incidence of West Nile virus and other VBZD.

270 Attwood, SW, Journal of Molluscan Studies, 1995. 61: p. 29-42, Kay, BH, et al., Journal of the American Mosquito Control Association, 1996. 12(3): p. 421-428, Maszle, DR, et al., Science of the Total Environment, 1998. 216(3): p. 193-203.

271 Vasconcelos, CH, et al., Igarss 2003: Ieee International Geoscience and Remote Sensing Symposium, Vols I - VII, Proceedings, 2003: p. 4567-4569, 4610, Yohannes, M, et al., Tropical Medicine & International Health, 2005. 10(12): p. 1274-1285.

272 LeGuenno, B, Arch Virol Suppl, 1997. 13: p. 191-199.

273 Brunkard, JM, et al., Emerging Infectious Diseases, 2007. 13(10): p. 1477-1483, Reiter, P, et al., Emerging Infectious Diseases, 2003. 9(1): p. 86-89.

Research Needs

Given the potential for significant increases in the burden of VBZD as a result of climate change, public health preparation is required, and research needs include:

* understanding of VBZD transmission cycles and the impact of ecological management and disruption on VBZD transmission, including the impact of new and intensified selective pressures due to climate change

* developing methods to detect, quantify, characterize, and monitor potential VBZD transmission associated with changes in terrestrial, ocean, coastal, and Great Lakes environments

* developing and validating models of VBZD ecology that link established datasets of VBZD disease transmission, identify relevant climate-related patterns, and integrate downscaled climate projections of likely impacts

* understanding of secondary effects of climate change such as increased malnutrition, conflict, and population displacement on VBZD, and evaluation of the effectiveness of prevention strategies

* enhancing research on the effectiveness of novel personal disease prevention methods including vaccines, repellents, bed nets, chemoproprophylaxis, and others[274]

* developing new pesticides aimed at controlling disease vectors that combine the qualities of specificity (affecting only the target arthropods), adjustable persistence through formulation (chemically labile but persistent for useful periods), environmental safety (no bioaccumulation or effect on non-target organisms), low susceptibility to resistance (through either inherent physiology or effective resistance management techniques), and application to creative control strategies

* enhancing existing public health surveillance infrastructure to include longitudinal surveillance focused on the periphery of endemic areas to detect range expansion and on ports of entry (airports, seaports) where vectors may penetrate after long-distance travel

* enhancing existing animal health surveillance (both domestic animals and wildlife) and early detection of emerging diseases of animal origin with particular emphasis on increased human to wildlife contact

274 Strickman, D, et al. 2009, Oxford ; New York: Oxford University Press. xviii, 323 p., [8] p. of plates.

- developing early warning systems that integrate public and animal health surveillance, risk assessments, and mitigation and adaptation strategies related to VBZD transmission

- enhancing research on risk communication and prevention strategies related to VBZD outbreak response including evaluation of their effectiveness

The research needs identified for VBZD include crosscutting issues and opportunities for leveraging co-benefits. Enhanced surveillance capacity is transferable to other health categories. Deeper understanding of the ecology of VBZD will enable understanding of other ecosystems, and improve our ability to preserve ecosystem services and limit ecosystem mismanagement. Developing mathematical models of VBZD ecology and linking these models with downscaled climate projections will generate novel modeling methodologies, as well as new methods in spatial epidemiology and mapping, and enhance existing public health workforce capacity. Research into risk communication and prevention strategies for VBZD can be applied to other health risks, both climate-related and otherwise. Novel strategies for application of vector control will benefit public health and infrastructure development in general. Because vector abatement efforts require organization that reaches multiple levels (household, farm), such efforts will form an interactive customer base for the application of environmental tools such as spatial analysis and monitoring to other environmental services such as building code enforcement, water standards, and sanitation, as well as provide additional resources for gathering operational data on the status of populations.

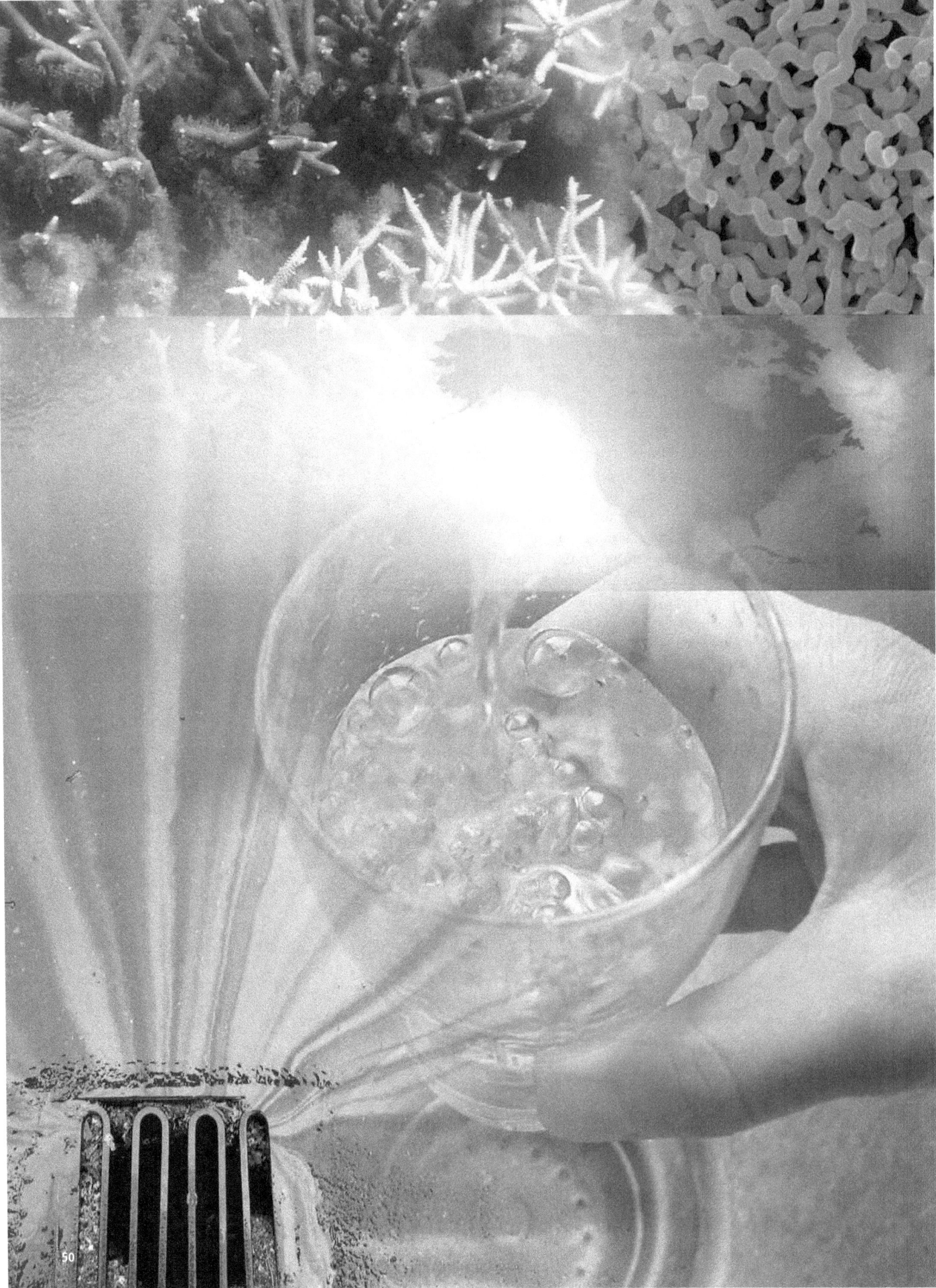

Waterborne Diseases

Waterborne diseases are caused by a wide variety of pathogenic microorganisms, biotoxins, and toxic contaminants found in the water we drink, clean with, play in, and are exposed to through other less direct pathways such as cooling systems. Waterborne microorganisms include protozoa that cause cryptosporidiosis, parasites that cause schistosomiasis, bacteria that cause cholera and legionellosis, viruses that cause viral gastroenteritis, amoebas that cause amoebic meningoencephalitis, and algae that cause neurotoxicity.[275] In the United States, the majority of waterborne disease is gastrointestinal, though waterborne pathogens affect most human organ systems and the epidemiology is dynamic. A recent shift has been seen in waterborne disease outbreaks from gastrointestinal toward respiratory infections such as that caused by *Legionella*, which lives in cooling ponds and is transmitted through air conditioning systems.[276] In addition to diarrheal disease, waterborne pathogens are implicated in other illnesses with immunologic, neurologic, hematologic, metabolic, pulmonary, ocular, renal and nutritional complications.[277] The World Health Organization estimates that 4.8% of the global burden of disease (as measured in disability-adjusted life years, or DALYs) and 3.7% of all mortality attributable to the environment is due to diarrheal disease.[278] Most of these diseases produce more serious symptoms and greater risk of death in children and pregnant women.[279]

For most waterborne pathogens in the United States, surveillance is spotty, diagnoses are not uniform, and our understanding of the impact of normal weather and climate variation on disease incidence, as well as illness and death burdens, is not firmly established. Impacts of any intensifying of climate events at local, regional, national, and global levels are a growing concern. Experts estimate that there is a high incidence of mild symptoms from waterborne pathogens and a relatively small, but not negligible mortality burden.[280]

275. Batterman, S., et al., Environ Health Perspect, 2009. 117(7): p. 1023-32.
276. Yoder, J., et al., MMWR Surveill Summ, 2008. 57(9): p. 39-62.
277. Meinhardt, PL, J Water Health, 2006. 4 Suppl 1: p. 27-34.
278. Mathers, C, et al. 2008, Geneva, Switzerland: World Health Organization. vii, 146 p.
279. Ibid.
280. Craun, GF, et al., J Water Health, 2006. 4 Suppl 2: p. 101-19.

RESEARCH HIGHLIGHT

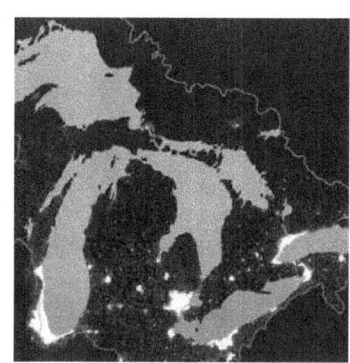

There is a clear association between increases in precipitation and outbreaks of waterborne disease, both domestically and globally. Climate change is expected to produce more frequent and severe extreme precipitation events worldwide. In the United States from 1948 to 1994, heavy rainfall correlated with more than half of the outbreaks of waterborne diseases.[1] Some of the largest outbreaks of waterborne disease in North America, particularly in the Great Lakes, have resulted after extreme rainfall events. For example, in May 2000, heavy rainfall in Walkerton, Ontario resulted in approximately 2,300 illnesses and seven deaths after the town's drinking water became contaminated with *E. coli* O157:H7 and *Campylobacter jejuni*.[2] There are 734 combined sewage and wastewater systems in and around the Great Lakes, with an estimated discharge of 850 billion gallons of untreated overflow water.[3] Using a suite of seven climate change models to project extreme precipitation events in the Great Lakes region, scientists have been able to estimate the potential impact of climate change on waterborne disease rates.[4] Their models predict more than 2.5 inches of rain in a single day will cause a combined sewer overflow into Lake Michigan, resulting in 50–100% more waterborne disease outbreaks in the region per year. Considering that the Great Lakes serves as the primary water source for over 40 million people and is surrounded by a number of large cities, both past events and these projections indicate a serious threat to public health in this region due to climate change alterations in the frequency of extreme precipitation.

1. Curriero, FC, et al., Am J Public Health, 2001. 91(8): p. 1194-9.
2. Hrudey, SE, et al., Water Science and Technology, 2003. 47(3): p. 7-14.
3. US Environmental Protection Agency, Report to Congress: Impacts and control of CSOs and SSOs. Office of Wastewater Management. 2004, US Environmental Protection Agency: Washington, DC.
4. Patz, JA, et al., Am J Prev Med, 2008. 35(5): p. 451-8.

Globally, the impact of waterborne diarrheal disease is high and expected to climb with climate change. Improving domestic surveillance is a high priority, as this would enhance epidemiologic characterization of the drivers of epidemic disease. In particular, weather and climate-related drivers are not well understood. Waterborne disease outbreaks are highly correlated with extreme precipitation events,[281] but this correlation is based on limited research and needs further investigation and confirmation. Prevention and treatment strategies for waterborne disease are well established throughout the developed world; climate change is not likely to greatly impact the efficacy of these strategies in the United States. However, climate change is very likely to increase global diarrheal disease incidence, and changes in the hydrologic cycle including increases in the frequency and intensity of extreme weather events and droughts may greatly complicate already inadequate prevention efforts. Enhanced understanding and reinvigorated global prevention efforts are very important.

Ocean-related diseases are those associated with direct contact with marine waters (aerosolized in some cases) or sediments (including beach sands), ingestion of contaminated seafood, or exposure to zoonotics.[282] Pathogenic microorganisms (bacteria, viruses, protozoa, and fungi) that may occur naturally in ocean, coastal, and Great Lakes waters, or as a result of sewage pollution and runoff, are the primary etiologic agents.[283] Human exposure to these agents may result in a variety of infectious diseases including serious wound and skin infections, diarrhea, respiratory effects, and others.[284] Research has concluded that the antibiotic resistant methicillin resistant *Staphylococcus aureus* (MRSA) is persistent in both fresh and seawater and could become waterborne if released into these waters in sufficient quantities.[285] While this has yet to emerge as a significant public health concern, the potential for recreational exposure is significant, as people make nearly one billion trips to the beach annually in the United States alone. In contrast to diarrheal disease, there are few effective preventive strategies for marine-based environmental exposures beyond

closing beaches to the public, and these areas need immediate additional research.

The effects of climate changes on the distribution and bioaccumulation of chemical contaminants in marine food webs are poorly understood and may be significant for vulnerable populations of humans and animals. The U.S. Climate Change Science Program (CCSP) reported a likely increase in the spread of waterborne pathogens depending on the pathogens' survival, persistence, habitat range, and transmission in a changing environment.[286] In one specific example, the CCSP noted the strong association between sea surface temperature and proliferation of many *Vibrio* species and suggested that rising temperatures would likely lead to increased occurrence of enteric disease associated with *Vibrio* bacteria (*V. cholerae, V. vulnificus,* and *V. parahaemolyticus)* in the United States, including the potential for the occurrence of cholera and wound infections. Further, recent findings demonstrate that pathogens that can pose disease risks to humans occur widely in marine vertebrates and regularly contaminate shellfish and aquacultured finfish.[287]

Impacts on Risk

Climate directly impacts the incidence of waterborne disease through effects on water temperature and precipitation frequency and intensity. These effects are pathogen and pollutant specific, and risks for human disease are markedly affected by local conditions, including regional water and sewage treatment capacities and practices. Domestic water treatment plants may be susceptible to climate change leading to human health risks. For example, droughts may cause problems with increased concentrations of effluent pathogens and overwhelm water treatment plants; aging water treatment plants are particularly at risk.[288] Urbanization of coastal regions may lead to additional nutrient, chemical, and pathogen loading in runoff.[289]

281 Curriero, FC, et al., Am J Public Health, 2001. 91(8): p. 1194-9.
282 Heaney, CD, et al., Am J Epidemiol, 2009. 170(2): p. 164-72.
283 Mos, L, et al., Environ Toxicol Chem, 2006. 25(12): p. 3110-7.
284 Stewart, JR, et al., Environ Health, 2008. 7 Suppl 2: p. S3.
285 Tolba, O, et al., Int J Hyg Environ Health, 2008. 211(3-4): p. 398-402.

286 Ebi, K, et al. In Analyses of the effects of global change on human health and welfare and human systems. A Report by the U.S. Climate Change Science Program and the Subcommittee on Global Change Research, J Gamble, et al., Editors. 2008. USEPA: Washington, D. C.
287 Moore, SK, et al., Environmental Health: A Global Access Science Source, 2008. 7(SUPPL. 2).
288 Kistemann, T, et al., Applied and Environmental Microbiology, 2002. 68(5): p. 2188-2197, Patz, JA, et al., Am J Prev Med, 2008. 35(5): p. 451-8, Senhorst, HAJ, et al., Water Science and Technology, 2005. 51(5): p. 53-59, Wilby, R, et al., Weather, 2005. 60(7): p. 206-211
289 Dwight, RH, et al., American Journal of Public Health, 2004. 94(4): p. 565-567, Dwight, RH, et al., Water Environment Research, 2002. 74(1): p. 82-90, Semenza, JC, et al., Lancet Infectious Diseases, 2009. 9(6): p. 365-375.

Our understanding of weather and climate impacts on specific pathogens is incomplete. Climate also indirectly impacts waterborne disease through changes in ocean and coastal ecosystems including changes in pH, nutrient and contaminant runoff, salinity, and water security. These indirect impacts are likely to result in degradation of fresh water available for drinking, washing food, cooking, and irrigation, particularly in developing and emerging economies where much of the population still uses untreated surface water from rivers, streams, and other open sources for these needs. Even in countries that treat water, climate-induced changes in the frequency and intensity of extreme weather events could lead to damage or flooding of water and sewage treatment facilities, increasing the risk of waterborne diseases. Severe outbreaks of cholera, in particular, have been directly associated with flooding in Africa and India.[290] A rise in sea level, combined with increasingly severe weather events, is likely to make flooding events commonplace worldwide. A 40 cm rise in sea level is expected to increase the average annual numbers of people affected by coastal storm surges from less than 50 million at present to nearly 250 million by 2080.[291]

Several secondary impacts are also a concern. Ecosystem degradation from climate change will likely result in pressure on agricultural productivity, crop failure, malnutrition, starvation, increasing population displacement, and resource conflict, all of which are predisposing factors for increased human susceptibility and increased risk of waterborne disease transmission due to surface water contamination with human waste and increased contact with such waters through washing and consumption.[292,293]

Climate change may also affect the distribution and concentrations of chemical contaminants in coastal and ocean waters, for example through release of chemical contaminants previously bound up in polar ice sheets or sediments, through changes in volume and composition of runoff from coastal and watershed development, or through changes in coastal and ocean goods and services. Both naturally occurring and pollution-related ocean health threats will likely be exacerbated by climate change.[294] Other climate-related environmental changes may impact marine food webs as well, such as pesticide runoff, leaching of arsenic, fluoride, and nitrates from fertilizers, and lead contamination of drinking and recreational waters through excess rainfall and flooding.

Mitigation and Adaptation

Alternative energy production, carbon sequestration, and water reuse and recycling are some of the mitigation and adaptation options that could have the greatest implications for human health. As with all technologies, the costs and benefits of each will need to be carefully considered and the most beneficial implemented.

The potential impacts of different mitigation strategies for waterborne illness depend on the strategy. For instance, increased hydroelectric power generation will have significant impacts on local ecologies where dams are built, often resulting in increased or decreased incidence of waterborne disease, as was the case with schistosomiasis (increase) and haematobium infection (decrease) after construction of the Aswan Dam in Egypt.[295] Other modes of electric power generation, including nuclear, consume large quantities of water and have great potential environmental impacts ranging from increased water scarcity to discharge of warmed effluent into local surface water bodies. Shifting to wind and solar power, however, will reduce demand on surface waters and, therefore, limit impacts on local water ecosystems and potentially reduce risks of waterborne diseases. The impacts on waterborne pathogen ecology of other geoengineering mitigation strategies, such as carbon sequestration, have the potential to be substantial but are currently largely unknown.[296] Thorough health impact and environmental impact assessments are necessary prior to implementation and widespread adoption of any novel mitigation technology.

There is also significant potential for adaptation activities to impact the ecology of waterborne infectious disease. Certain adaptation strategies are likely to have a beneficial impact on water quality; for instance, protecting wetlands to reduce damage from severe storms.

290 Sidley, P, BMJ, 2008. 336(7642): p. 471; Sur, D, et al., Indian J Med Res, 2000. 112: p. 178-82.
291 Ford, TE, et al., Emerging Infectious Diseases, 2009. 15(9): p. 1341-1346.
292 Shultz, A, et al., American Journal of Tropical Medicine and Hygiene, 2009. 80(4): p. 640-645.
293 Diaz, JH, Am J Disaster Med, 2007. 2(1): p. 33-42.

294 Sandifer, P, et al., Interagency oceans and human health research implementation plan: a prescription for the future. 2007, Interagency Working Group on Harmful Algal Blooms, Hypoxia and Human Health of the Joint Subcommittee on Ocean Science and Technology: Washington, DC, USA.
295 Abdel-Wahab, MF, et al., Lancet, 1979. 2(8136): p. 242-4.
296 White, CM, et al., Energy & Fuels, 2005. 19(3): p. 659-724.

Under drought conditions, water reuse or the use of water sources that may be of lower quality is likely to increase.[297] Local water recycling and so-called grey-water reuse, as well as urban design strategies to increase green space and reduce runoff, may result in slower rates of water table depletion and reduce the impact of extreme precipitation events in urban areas where runoff is concentrated.

Other adaptation efforts may have both positive and negative effects. For instance, if the response to increasingly frequent and severe heat waves is widespread adoption of air conditioning, the associated increase in electricity demand will require additional power, which in turn could impact water availability and regional water ecology. In parts of the developing world, changing weather patterns and decreased food availability could lead to increased desertification, or at the least the need for more above-ground irrigation. If such projects are implemented in areas where parasitic diseases such as schistosomiasis are prevalent without close attention to potential ecosystem impacts, there may be changes in regional parasite transport and associated increases or decreases in human exposure.

Climate-induced changes to coastal ecosystems are poorly understood, especially with regard to ecosystem goods and services related to human health and well being, and ocean and coastal disease threats.[298] Interactions among climate change factors such as rising temperature, extreme weather events, inundation, ocean acidification, and changes in precipitation and runoff with coastal development, aquacultural practices, and other water use issues need to be studied.

Research Needs

The extent to which the United States is vulnerable to increased risk of waterborne diseases and ocean-related illness due to climate change has not been adequately addressed.[299] Research needs include:

- understanding the likelihood and potential magnitude of waterborne disease outbreaks due to climate change including increases in the frequency and intensity of precipitation, temperature changes, extreme weather events, and storm surges

- researching the vulnerability of water systems to sewer overflow or flooding caused by extreme weather events, especially in water systems where there is already considerable water reuse; and examining the impacts of other water reuse and recycling strategies

- understanding how toxins, pathogens, and chemicals in land-based runoff and water overflow interact synergistically and with marine species, especially those important for human consumption, and the potential health risks of changing water quality

- developing means of identifying sentinel species for waterborne disease and understanding of how they may provide early warning of human health threats

- developing or improving vaccines, antibiotics and other preventive strategies to prevent and reduce the health consequences of waterborne disease on a global basis

- improving understanding of harmful algal blooms including their initiation, development, and termination, as well as the exact nature of the toxins associated with them

297 Corwin, DL, et al., J Environ Qual, 2008. 37(5 Suppl): p. S1-7.

298 United States. Congress. Senate. Committee on Commerce Science and Transportation. 2003, Washington: U.S. G.P.O. ii. 8 p.

299 Frumkin, H, et al., American Journal of Public Health, 2008. 98(3): p. 435-445. Ebi, K, et al. In Analyses of the effects of global change on human health and welfare and human systems. A Report by the U.S. Climate Change Science Program and the Subcommittee on Global Change Research, J Gamble, et al., Editors. 2008, USEPA: Washington, D. C. Sandifer, P, et al., Interagency oceans and human health research implementation plan: a prescription for the future. 2007, Interagency Working Group on Harmful Algal Blooms, Hypoxia and Human Health of the Joint Subcommittee on Ocean Science and Technology: Washington, DC, USA.

- conducting epidemiologic studies on the occurrence and severity of ocean-related diseases among humans, especially high risk populations, in relation to climate change

- evaluating and monitoring exposures and health risks of chemical contaminants likely to be increasingly released and mobilized due to climate change

- improving methods to detect, quantify, and forecast ocean-related health threats including improved surveillance and monitoring of disease-causing agents in coastal waters; in marine organisms (especially seafood), aerosols, and sediments; and in exposed human populations

- assessing the capacity of the nation's public health infrastructure to detect and respond to increased waterborne disease incidence, and developing training and evaluation tools to address identified gaps

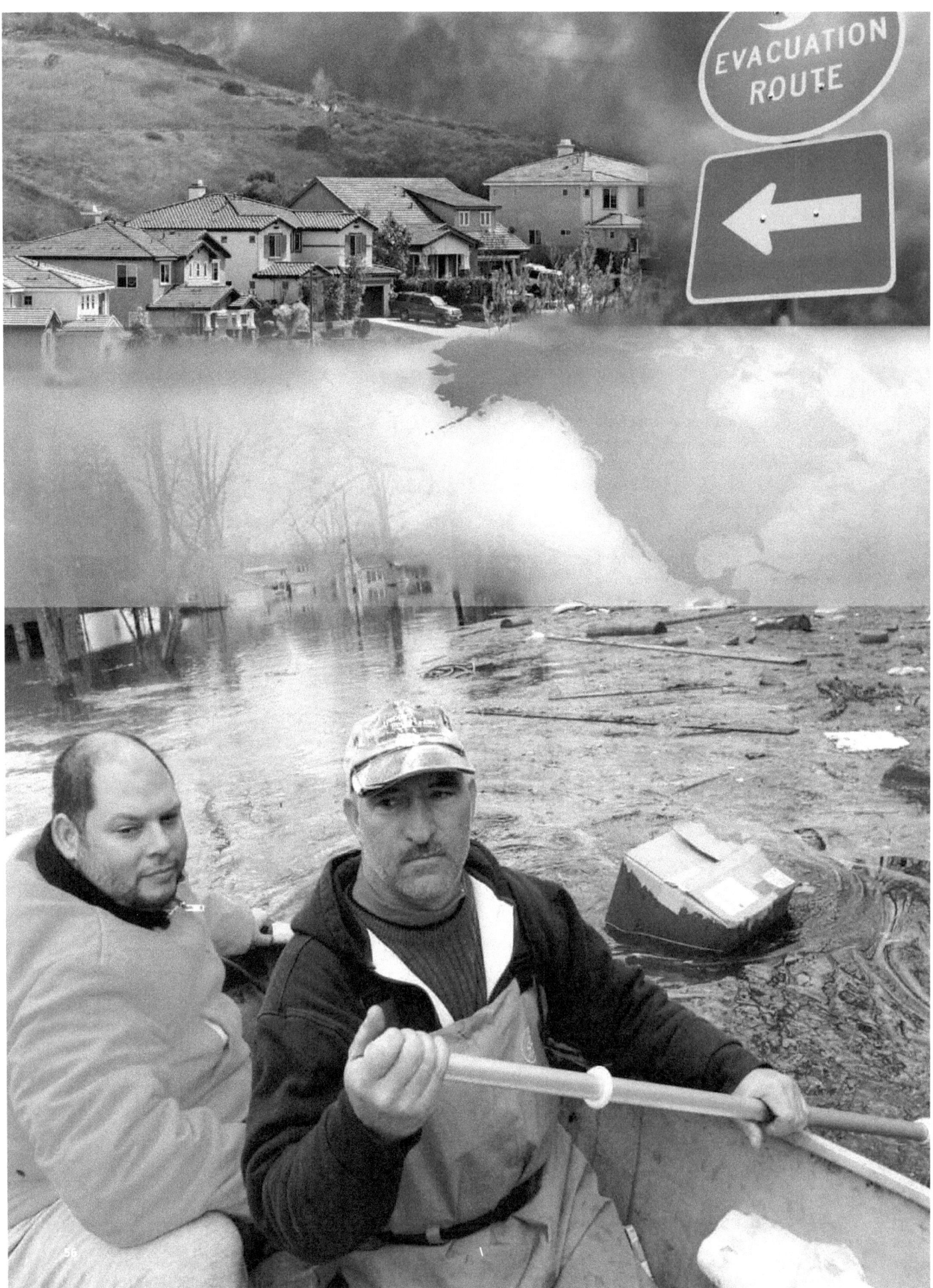

Weather-Related Morbidity and Mortality

The United States experiences a variety of extreme weather events ranging from hurricanes and floods to blizzards and drought. Many of these events cause severe infrastructure damage and lead to significant morbidity and mortality. From 1940 to 2005, hurricanes caused approximately 4,300 deaths and flooding caused 7,000 deaths, primarily from injuries and drowning.[300] Climate change is expected to increase the frequency and intensity of some extreme weather events, including floods, droughts, and heat waves, though how these events will manifest on a regional level is uncertain.[301] The health impacts of these extreme weather events can be severe, and include both direct impacts such as death and mental health effects, and indirect impacts such as population displacement and waterborne disease outbreaks such as the 1993 Milwaukee cryptosporidium outbreak caused by flooding that sickened an estimated 400,000 people.[302, 303]

The populations most at risk from such extreme events also are growing, particularly as a result of increased coastal development, as recent flooding events and hurricanes have shown. Sea-level rise associated with climate change will amplify the threat from storm surge associated with extreme weather events in coastal areas.[304] Other areas, such as the Southwest, are at risk for decreased agricultural productivity due to increased drought and possible compromise of potable water supplies due to flooding from heavy precipitation events.[305] Given the increased incidence of extreme weather events and the increasing number of people at risk, research in this area is an immediate and significant need. Preparation has a significant impact on outcomes of extreme weather events. Poor preparedness and response to Hurricane Katrina led to increased morbidity and mortality, as well as economic costs associated with recovery, which were estimated to be in excess of $150 billion.[306] By increasing research funding related to extreme weather events,

increased preparedness levels could lower costs and minimize morbidity and mortality from future events.

Impacts on Risk

A changing climate coupled with changing demographics is expected to magnify the already significant adverse effects of extreme weather on public health. For example, the intensity and frequency of precipitation events in the United States have increased over the past 100 years in many locations.[307] In the Midwest and Northeastern United States, heavy rainfall events (defined as those in excess of 1 inch of rainfall) have increased by as much as 100%, and recent flooding events, such as the June 2008 flooding in the Midwest, have caused billions of dollars of damage and significant loss of life.[308] In line with this observed trend, there is a projected increase in intensity of precipitation events in some areas of the country, particularly in the Northeast, which has experienced a 67% increase in the amount of heavy precipitation events in the past 50 years.[309, 310] Precipitation extremes also are expected to increase more than the mean. Regional variability appears to be increasing so that even though extreme precipitation events will become more common, some areas will concurrently experience drought, especially in the northeast and southwest.[311]

The intensity of extreme precipitation events is projected to increase with future warming.[312] This could limit the ability to capture and store water in reservoirs, leading to flash flooding events. Climate variability resulting from naturally occurring climate phenomena such as El Niño, La Niña, and global monsoons, are associated with extreme weather events around the globe.[313] El Niño and La Niña conditions lead to changes in the patterns of tropical rainfall

300 Ashley, ST, et al., Journal of Applied Meteorology and Climatology, 2008. 47(3): p. 805-818. National Weather Service, Summary of Natural Hazard Statistics for 2007 in the United States. 2007: Washington.
301 Greenough, G, et al., Environmental Health Perspectives, 2001. 109: p. 191-198. Trenberth, KE, et al., Bulletin of the American Meteorological Society, 2003. 84(9): p. 1205-+.
302 Mac Kenzie, WR, et al., N Engl J Med, 1994. 331(3): p. 161-7.
303 Greenough, G, et al., Environmental Health Perspectives, 2001. 109: p. 191-198. Mills, DM, Journal of Occupational and Environmental Medicine, 2009. 51(1): p. 26-32. Verger, P, et al., Journal of Exposure Analysis and Environmental Epidemiology, 2003. 13(6): p. 436-442.
304 Karl, T, et al., Weather and climate extremes in a changing climate regions of focus: North America, Hawaii, Caribbean, and U.S. Pacific Islands, in Synthesis and assessment product 3.3. 2008, U.S. Climate Change Science Program: Washington, DC. p. x, 162 p.
305 Ibid.
306 Burton, M, et al., Hurricane Katrina: Preliminary estimates of commercial and public sector damages. 2005, Center for Business and Economic Research, Marshall University: Huntington, WV.

307 Karl, T, et al. 2009. New York: Cambridge University Press. Kunkel, KE, Natural Hazards, 2003. 29(2): p. 291-305.
308 Black, H, Environmental Health Perspectives, 2008. 116(9): p. A390-+. Kunkel, KE, et al., Journal of Climate, 1999. 12(8): p. 2515-2527.
309 Kunkel, KE, Natural Hazards, 2003. 29(2): p. 291-305, Balling, RC, et al., Natural Hazards, 2003. 29(2): p. 103-112, Groisman, PY, et al., Climatic Change, 1999. 42(1): p. 243-283.
310 Meehl, GAas, T. F. and Collins, W. D. and Friedlingstein, A. T. and Gaye, A. T. and Gregory, J. M. and Kitoh, A. and Knutti, R. and Murphy, J. M. and Noda, A. and Raper, S. C. B. and Watterson, I. G. and Weaver, A. J. and Zhao, Z. in Climate change 2007 : the physical science basis : contribution of Working Group I to the Fourth Assessment Report of the Intergovernmental Panel on Climate Change, S Solomon, et al., Editors. 2007, Cambridge University Press: Cambridge ; New York. p. 747-845.
311 Christensen, JH, et al. ibid. Hayhoe, K, et al., Climate Dynamics, 2007. 28(4): p. 381-407, Milly, PCD, et al., Nature, 2005. 438(7066): p. 347-350.
312 Meehl, GAas, T. F. and Collins, W. D. and Friedlingstein, A. T. and Gaye, A. T. and Gregory, J. M. and Kitoh, A. and Knutti, R. and Murphy, J. M. and Noda, A. and Raper, S. C. B. and Watterson, I. G. and Weaver, A. J. and Zhao, Z. in Climate change 2007 : the physical science basis : contribution of Working Group I to the Fourth Assessment Report of the Intergovernmental Panel on Climate Change, S Solomon, et al., Editors. 2007, Cambridge University Press: Cambridge ; New York. p. 747-845.
313 Karl, T, et al., Weather and climate extremes in a changing climate regions of focus: North America, Hawaii, Caribbean, and U.S. Pacific Islands, in Synthesis and assessment product 3.3. 2008, U.S. Climate Change Science Program: Washington, DC. p. x, 162 p.

and in the weather patterns in mid-latitudes, including changes in the frequency and intensity of weather extremes. El Niño is also projected to increase in both frequency and intensity as the climate warms, though there is uncertainty about the relative frequency of El Niño and La Niña in the future. Increased precipitation associated with stronger El Niño events would affect the Western United States, particularly California, the Pacific Northwest, and the Gulf Coast more than other regions of the country.[314]

Heavy precipitation events will be highly variable in magnitude, duration, and geographic location. Increased variability in weather and climate extremes is difficult to predict, and will impact the ability of human systems to manage for and adapt to heavy precipitation and flooding events. An observed divergence of precipitation patterns has lead to increased variability in the amount of precipitation per event, resulting in both extreme amounts of precipitation, as well as abnormally small precipitation events.[315] These effects have already been observed globally. A study in Germany found that winter storms from 1901 to 2000 showed an increasing trend of precipitation events both exceeding the 95th percentile and falling below the 5th percentile; while from 1956 to 2004 the Dongxiang River in China became increasingly likely to be at either extreme flood flow or abnormally low-flow.[316]

The current evidence is insufficient to determine if the frequency of tropical cyclones in the Atlantic Basin will change. The observed frequency of tropical cyclones in the Atlantic Basin has increased since the mid-1990s, though the numbers are not unprecedented and must be reconciled with active multi-decadal periods of the past, such as the 1950s and 1960s.[317] Increases in sea surface temperature and decreases in wind shear may lead to more intense Atlantic hurricanes, though some models also show a decrease in the number of intense hurricanes in the Atlantic Basin.

The spatial distribution of hurricanes also is likely to change, with storm surges becoming more damaging in areas unaccustomed to facing large hurricanes. The combination of sea-level rise with increasing storm intensity could lead to significant destruction of coastal

infrastructure and more costly hurricanes.[318] In addition, flooding and coastal changes could lead to ecosystem changes such as loss of wetlands that could indirectly impact human health. Hurricane track forecasting and modeling methods have improved, and mortality rates for major storms have declined over time, but the combination of increased coastal population density, increased intensity of tropical storms, and sea-level rise will result in significantly increased risk going forward.[319]

Some models show that what were 20-year floods in 1860 in the United Kingdom are now 5-year floods; even greater impacts are expected in tropical regions.[320] In the United States, large floods are more frequent now than at the beginning of the 20th century.[321] Monsoon-related flooding results in damaged infrastructure, increased disease, and loss of life. During El Niño, areas includig Indonesia, southern Africa, northeastern Australia, and northeastern Brazil usually experience extensive periods of dry weather and warmer-than-average temperatures.[322] These conditions have historically resulted in a variety of adverse effects, such as mudslides, forest fires and resulting increased air pollution, mass migrations, and famines.[323]

Mitigation and Adaptation

Climate change mitigation includes activities that reduce greenhouse gas emissions. Important sources include land use changes, transport, energy production, and buildings. Some proposed mitigation strategies to reduce the occurrence of extreme weather events could impact human health. A reduction in personal automobile usage is one way to lower carbon emissions. However, a greater reliance on pubic transportation could either improve or reduce the ability to quickly evacuate a city prior to a severe weather event, depending on how it is managed. Mitigation activities related to land use may have other health impacts; anthropogenic reforestation, when combined with shifting weather patterns, could provide habitats for zoonotic and vectorborne diseases while reducing land available for agricultural uses. It is difficult to adequately evaluate the likely health impacts of various mitigation strategies, though Health Impact Assessments are proving a very useful public health tool for this purpose.

314 Ibid, Easterling, DR, et al., Science, 2000. 289(5487): p. 2068-2074.
315 Jentsch, A, et al., Comptes Rendus Geoscience, 2008. 340(9-10): p. 621-628, Christensen, JH, et al. In Climate change 2007 : the physical science basis : contribution of Working Group I to the Fourth Assessment Report of the Intergovernmental Panel on Climate Change, S Solomon, et al., Editors. 2007, Cambridge University Press: Cambridge ; New York. p. 747-845.
316 Tromel, S, et al., Theoretical and Applied Climatology, 2007. 87(1-4): p. 29-39, Wang, W, et al., Hydrology and Earth System Sciences, 2008. 12(1): p. 207-221
317 Karl, T, et al., Weather and climate extremes in a changing climate regions of focus: North America, Hawaii, Caribbean, and U.S. Pacific Islands, in Synthesis and assessment product 3.3. 2008, U.S. Climate Change Science Program: Washington, DC. p. x, 162 p. Henderson-Sellers, A, et al., Bulletin of the American Meteorological Society, 1998. 79(1): p. 19-38, Knutson, T, et al. in Culture Extremes and Society. 2008, Cambridge University Press: Cambridge.

318 Meehl, GAas, T. F. and Collins, W. D. and Friedlingstein, A. T. and Gaye, A. T. and Gregory, J. M. and Kitoh, A. and Knutti, R. and Murphy, J. M. and Noda, A. and Raper, S. C. B. and Watterson, I. G. and Weaver, A. J. and Zhao, Z. in Climate change 2007 : the physical science basis : contribution of Working Group I to the Fourth Assessment Report of the Intergovernmental Panel on Climate Change, S Solomon, et al., Editors. 2007, Cambridge University Press: Cambridge ; New York. p. 747-845.
319 Rappaport, EN, et al., Weather and Forecasting, 2009. 24(2): p. 395-419.
320 Allen, MR, et al., Nature, 2002. 419(6903): p. 224-+.
321 Trenberth, KE, et al., Bulletin of the American Meteorological Society, 2003. 84(9): p. 1205-+, Milly, PCD, et al., Nature, 2005. 438(7066): p. 347-350.
322 Karl, T, et al., Weather and climate extremes in a changing climate regions of focus: North America, Hawaii, Caribbean, and U.S. Pacific Islands, in Synthesis and assessment product 3.3. 2008, U.S. Climate Change Science Program: Washington, DC. p. x, 162 p.
323 Planton, S, Medecine Et Maladies Infectieuses, 1999. 29(5): p. 267-276.

There are several adaptation strategies for extreme weather events that have proven effective, including early warning systems, zoning and planning to avoid building in at-risk areas, reinforcing the built environment against hazardous weather events, and evacuation planning. While some strategies may be costly, they can be implemented over extended periods of time, defraying their costs. However, adaptation could be more difficult in some of the most heavily affected areas. For example, the population of many cities along the relatively high-risk U.S. Eastern seaboard has been growing in recent years and this growth is likely to continue. High population growth, typically associated with concentrations of critical infrastructure, in areas vulnerable to storm surges and sea-level rise will make adaptation difficult. Moreover, some adaptation activities intended to preserve existing infrastructure, such as building levees and other flood control measures, may have adverse ecological impacts and be prohibitively expensive. Alternatively, measures to fortify natural barriers to flooding and erosion and to buffer storm surge, such as wetlands and tidal marshes, will decrease the magnitude of adverse exposures and maintain associated ecosystem services such as food production and waste assimilation, thereby realizing potential co-benefits of climate change adaptation.

Research Needs

Due to the complexity of climate change and the health effects associated with climate variability and extreme weather, research needs in this area are diverse, and include:

- exploring the impact of extreme precipitation events on waterborne disease, particularly cholera, and on the ecology of vectorborne and zoonotic disease

- improving understanding of extreme weather events associated with naturally occurring climate phenomena such as El Niño, La Niña, and monsoons, and their impacts on human health

- assessing the ability of health care systems to respond to extreme weather events and provide uninterrupted access to and delivery of health care services under a variety of scenarios

- improving understanding of how to anticipate and address food security and nutrition issues after extreme weather events, domestically and globally

- improving understanding of how to anticipate and address water quality and availability concerns associated with extreme weather events, domestically and globally

- developing strategies for linking health databases[324] with real-time monitoring and prospective assessment of weather, climate, geospatial, and exposure data[325] in order to better characterize the health impacts of extreme weather events

- improving the predictive power of probabilistic modeling of health effects of extreme events such as droughts, wildfires, and floods

- enhancing predictability, modeling, and ongoing assessment of the effects of climate variability and change (seasonal-to-interannual and decadal) on extreme events and correlation with short- and long-term health outcomes

- developing and validating downscaling techniques from global climate models to provide regional information for health early warning systems

- transitioning research advances into operational products and decision support tools for health early warning systems

- evaluating and improving the effectiveness of health alert warning systems and other health system risk communication tools such as evacuation protocols and National Disaster Management System activation, particularly for high-risk populations

- expanding research on prevention and preparedness for extreme weather events including development of disaster planning tools such as data and communication systems for public health and emergency care, including enhanced access to medical records and capabilities across hospitals on a regional level

- evaluating and developing new funding and reinsurance strategies and policies for disaster relief and rebuilding infrastructure

Weather related research intersects with several other areas of climate change research. Examples include waterborne and vectorborne illness following floods and hurricane storm surges, as well as post-traumatic stress disorder and related mental effects that can result from personal tragedy and displacement after extreme weather events. Studies of marine ecosystems and associated health impacts also overlap with extreme weather studies. Research in health communications and early warning systems is clearly applicable to periods proceeding and following weather disasters, as well as disaster preparedness and critical infrastructure development and protection

---

324 such as the databases maintained by the National Center for Health Statistics
325 such as the databases included in the Global Earth Observation System of Systems Initiative and those maintained by the US EPA and NOAA

Synthesis and Recommendations

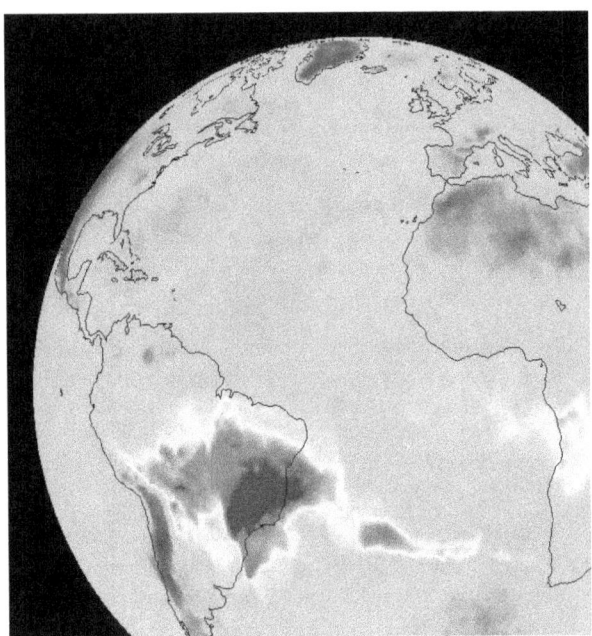

There is abundant evidence that human activities are altering the earth's climate and that climate change will have significant health impacts both domestically and globally. While all of the changes associated with this process are not predetermined, the actions we take today will certainly help to shape our environment in the decades to come. Some degree of climate change is unavoidable, and we must adapt to its associated health effects; however, aggressive mitigation actions can significantly blunt the worst of the expected exposures. Still, there will be effects on the health of people in the United States, some of which are probably already underway. As great as the domestic risks to U.S. public health are, the global risks are even greater.

Climate change and health issues transcend national borders, and climate change health impacts in other countries are likely to affect health in the United States as well. Famine, drought, extreme weather events, and regional conflicts—all likely consequences of climate change—are some of the factors that increase the incidence and severity of disease, as well as contributing to other adverse health impacts, making it imperative to address climate change-related decision making at local, regional, national, and global levels. The complicated interplay of these and other factors must be considered in determining the scope and focus of both basic and applied research on climate change and health.

There are significant research needs to help direct adaptation activities and inform mitigation choices going forward. Such needs include integrating climate science with health science; integrating environmental, public health, and marine and wildlife surveillance; applying climate and meteorological observations to real-time public health issues; and down-scaling long-term climate models to estimate human exposure risks and burden of disease. Integrated data systems should incorporate a breadth of environmental parameters, as well as sociodemographic parameters such as population, income, and education.

Several overarching themes emerged during the creation of this document including: systems and complexity, risk communication and public health education, co-benefits of mitigation and adaptation strategies, and urgency and scope. These are discussed below.

Systems and Complexity. The complicated links between human and natural systems need to be better understood so public health agencies can develop evidence-based prevention strategies and the health care community can pursue secondary controls and respond to health incidents when prevention is not effective. Research on these links should focus not only on the direct health effects of climate change but also on the complex relationships between different exposure pathways and health risks. For example, people with compromised immune systems because of persistent organic pollutant exposure are likely to be at greater risk of infection and death from vectorborne, waterborne, and foodborne pathogens and disease. Similarly, people with respiratory illnesses such as asthma and chronic obstructive pulmonary disease are far more likely to suffer distress and hospitalization during extreme heat events, dust storms, or high pollen events than healthy people. Thus, the structure of basic research on health impacts should address the combined effects of multiple environmental changes and stressors, some caused by climate change and some by other factors, facilitating a robust public health and health care response.

Given the fundamental importance of ecosystems in climate change impacts and the significant roles that environmental factors play in human health, climate change and health research should also focus on the complex interplay between risk, location, and environmental conditions. Vulnerability and resilience to climate change health effects are both heavily determined by locality. A huge amount of diverse information will be needed at all governance levels (local, regional, national, global). Understanding local needs will be of greatest importance, given that effective adaptation strategies likely will not be universally applicable to all locations. However, there is also a need to identify common elements of strategies that may be generalized from one community to another. In addition, research is needed on how to identify common features of locales that will help identify them as having similar responses to climate change, how to determine and develop optimal strategies for interventions, and how to develop and implement communication tools that will effectively help communities respond to their particular situation.

Risk Communication and Public Health Education. Knowledge is one of the most strategic tools in reducing health problems in any environment; it allows us to understand what is harmful, why, and possibly how to avoid such harm. Research is critical, but knowledge that is not effectively communicated to appropriate audiences is wasted. Knowledge of the health impacts associated with climate change will have limited value without effective communication and education strategies to increase public awareness and understanding of the specific risks involved and the complexity of the issues. Communication with particularly vulnerable individuals and populations, as well as with health care professionals and public health officials tasked with protecting communities, is itself deserving of further research. For example, public health agencies already warn people with pulmonary diseases to avoid lengthy exposure outdoors on days of high ozone. Such warning systems might be more effective if delivered through multiple channels and tailored to individual health risks. Warnings on other harmful environmental exposures such as high pollen concentrations and extreme heat events should be expanded in geographic scope. For at-risk patients, warnings could be integrated into hospital and clinic discharge instructions or distributed with medications to more effectively prevent exacerbations of environmentally sensitive disease. Public health professionals need to be highly vigilant for opportunities to increase the range and impact of early warning systems on vulnerable populations. As our health care system is increasingly integrated and preventive health activities become more robust, there will be ever more opportunities to prevent adverse health effects associated with harmful environmental exposures. Risk communication efforts need to be culturally sensitive to provide appropriate and effective guidance, and potential interventions require testing and evaluation before they are implemented.

Mitigation and Adaptation. Considerable discussion currently focuses on identifying mitigation strategies that balance the economic costs of emission reductions (both direct mitigation costs and costs associated with loss of productivity) with the costs of environmental degradation from continuing business as usual. Examples of mitigation technologies include electric cars, alternative fuels, and green urban development. Cost-benefit evaluations typically express costs in economic terms rather than in terms of human morbidity and mortality, though these health impacts can be substantial. Many mitigation and adaptation strategies reach across health endpoints and may be both beneficial and problematic for a wide array of diseases.

Climate change health impacts are complicated and not always intuitive or unidirectional. For example, reducing reliance on fossil fuels in the transportation sector will substantially reduce CO_2 emissions, which over time will reduce the effects of climate change on human health. Thus, consideration of the costs of emissions reductions should include reduced health cost due to effective mitigation. Failing to mitigate also carries additional health consequences beyond those associated with climate change itself. For example, reducing vehicular emissions improves air quality, which may lessen incidences of effects such as airway diseases and irritations, cardiovascular disease, and cancer. However, further research, including life cycle analyses of batteries and other technologies, and human exposure to novel emission mixtures, is needed to avoid unintended negative consequences. If we choose not to reduce greenhouse gas emissions from transportation, levels of air pollution generated by vehicles will remain high and the cardiovascular, respiratory,

and cancer morbidity and mortality associated with vehicular air pollution will continue and probably increase. This example illustrates the importance of understanding the potential co-benefits of climate change mitigation efforts so that optimal strategies can be implemented. Basic research on health and environmental factors and implementation research to develop new models and paradigms for burden-of-disease calculations are needed to allow for a careful use of health and economic cost indicators in the same evaluation. Health impact assessments are an important tool for evaluating the health impacts, both positive and negative, of possible mitigation strategies prior to widespread implementation.

Similarly, there is considerable need for study of broader adaptation issues that will affect many different groups. Examples of adaptation include use of air conditioning, weather alerts, and increased numbers of medical facilities. Of key interest are the health effects of adaptation practices in food, water, and chemical use. For example, regional water shortages will cause a greater intensity of recycling and reuse of water, with resulting increases in risks of human exposure to waterborne pollutants and pathogens. The genetic modification of plants to withstand altered environments and use less water could introduce changes in the allergenicity or toxicity of foods that are currently considered harmless. And use of pesticides whose residues may be harmful to both current and future generations may increase as a way of adapting to the effects of increasing temperatures and changing precipitation patterns that affect crop yields. Other adaptation efforts may have important health co-benefits that need to be identified. For example, adaptation efforts focusing on urban design, such as increasing urban albedo through green roofs, increasing urban tree cover, reducing the size of the urban heat island through compact development, and decreasing impervious surface runoff through use of permeable paving surfaces have been shown to have multiple co-benefits.

By no means a comprehensive list, the strategies discussed above illustrate the diversity in mitigation and adaptation possibilities, and it should be noted that many new ideas and options are being developed. As with all emerging technologies, it is important to holistically examine their effects on health, both positive and negative, so that the best options for society can be identified and adopted.

Scope and Urgency. The necessary research on climate change health impacts, the health effects of mitigation, and development of appropriate adaptation strategies will not occur spontaneously and cannot occur in isolation. To be successful, an overarching research program needs to be integrated, focused, interdisciplinary, supported, and sustainable, yet flexible enough to adjust to new information and broad enough to cover the very diverse components described in this document. The effort must also be multinational, multiagency, and multidisciplinary, bringing together the strengths of all partners. The effort also must promote user-driven research that closely aligns future research directions with the needs of decision makers by facilitating multi-directional dialogue among information producers, providers, and end users. This research will require capacity building in a number of areas, especially in climate sciences and disease and ecosystem surveillance necessary to support the health sciences as they grapple with these issues. Finally, both the efforts and the outcomes need to be evaluated using clear metrics that are linked to assessment questions and outcome indicators to ensure they are valid, effective, and achieve the desired goals.

Natural systems adapt to environmental changes or they fail. Climate change threatens many of the natural and built systems that protect and preserve our nation's health. The infrastructure that we have put in place to protect health and provide well being in the United States is extremely diverse and includes hospitals, clinics, public health agencies, trained personnel, roads and transportation systems, the electrical grid, water treatment systems, and many other components. Threats to these systems from climate change range from damage to natural and built physical infrastructure to damage to intangible organizational structures (human and social capital) that are required to maintain resilience to environmental threats. Climate change could have grave impacts on public health systems if they are not appropriately strengthened. Research into the vulnerability of these systems will be critical to identifying areas most in need of attention, avoiding mistakes, limiting human suffering, and ultimately saving lives.

Summary Statement

Humans have successfully adapted to environmental change over time, from evolving natural physiological responses to the use of science, technology, and knowledge to improve our lives and advance our health. From the dawn of the industrial age, people have made great strides in improving health, and enjoy a markedly improved quality of life. However, these improvements have come at a cost that must now be understood and addressed. Climate change will force humans to negotiate with their changing environment as never before to find ways to reshape it both for short-term protection and long-term alleviation of health consequences.

There is no doubt that we have the capacity to find ways to avoid many of the worst health effects of climate change, and indeed, given the universality and potential magnitude of such effects, we have an ethical imperative to do so. The research needs described in this document should guide the process, helping us to develop the proper tools and make informed choices that will ultimately result in better health and better lives for the citizens of the United States and of the world.

Interagency Working Group on Climate Change and Health

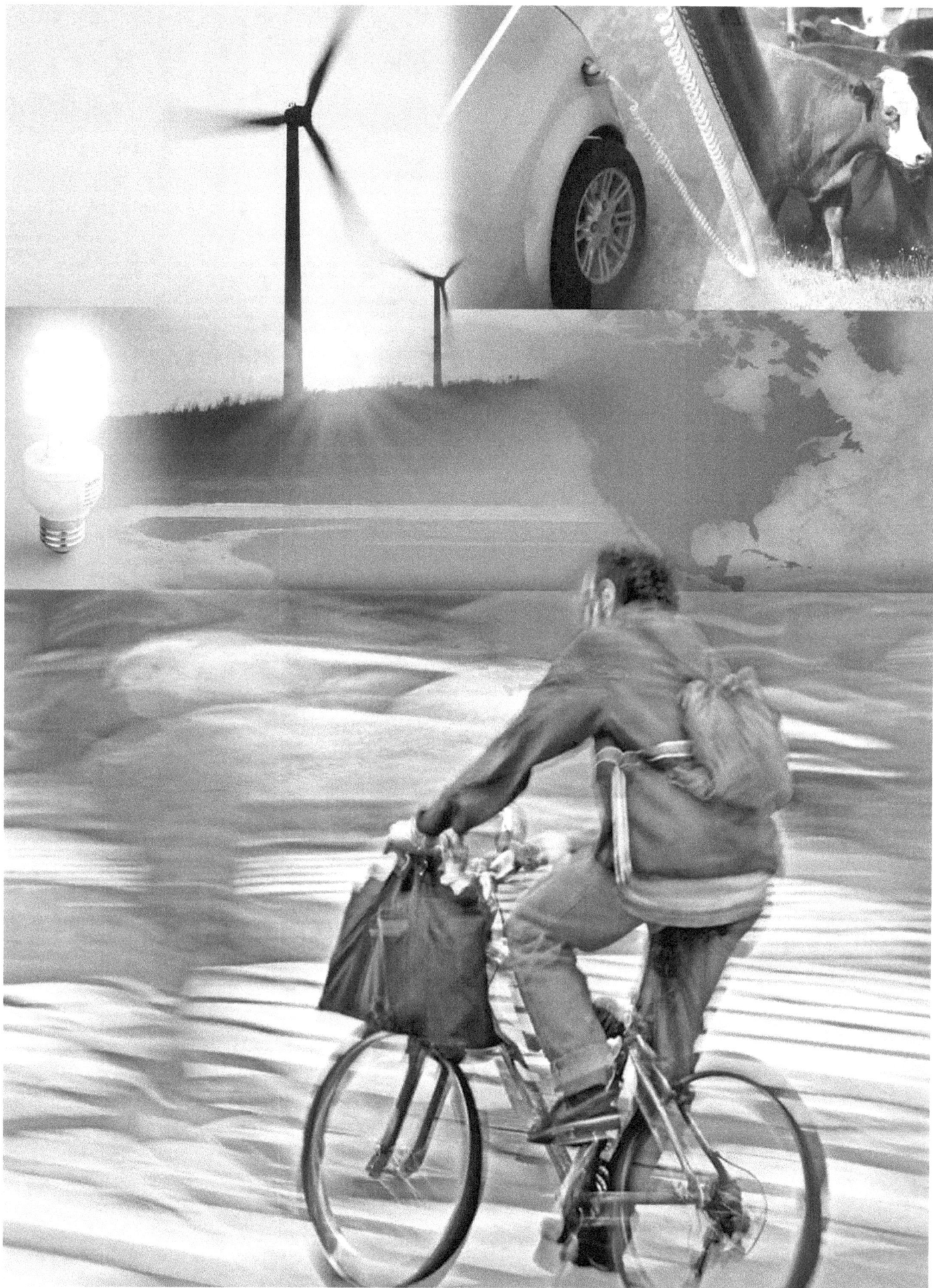

Bibliography

Aagaard-Tillery, K.M., *et al., Developmental origins of disease and determinants of chromatin structure: maternal diet modifies the primate fetal epigenome.* Journal of Molecular Endocrinology, 2008. **41**(2): p. 91-102.

Abdel-Wahab, M.F., *et al., Changing pattern of schistosomiasis in Egypt 1935—79.* Lancet, 1979. **2**(8136): p. 242-4.

Abraham, W.M., *et al., Effects of inhaled brevetoxins in allergic airways: toxin-allergen interactions and pharmacologic intervention.* Environmental Health Perspectives, 2005. **113**(5): p. 632-637.

Adler, P. and W. Wills, *The history of arthropod-borne human disease in South Carolina.* American Entomologist, 2003. **49**: p. 216-228.

Ahn, Y.H., *et al., Application of satellite infrared data for mapping of thermal plume contamination in coastal ecosystem of Korea.* Marine Environmental Research, 2006. **61**(2): p. 186-201.

al-Harthi, S.S., *et al., Non-invasive evaluation of cardiac abnormalities in heat stroke pilgrims.* Int J Cardiol, 1992. **37**(2): p. 151-4.

Albrecht, G., *et al., Solastalgia: the distress caused by environmental change.* Australasian Psychiatry, 2007. **15**: p. S95-S98.

Allen, M.R. and W.J. Ingram, *Constraints on future changes in climate and the hydrologic cycle.* Nature, 2002. **419**(6903): p. 224-+.

Altevogt, B.M., S.L. Hanson, and A.I. Leshner, *Autism and the environment: Challenges and opportunities for research.* Pediatrics, 2008. **121**(6): p. 1225-1229.

American Heart Association. *Cardiovascular disease cost, 2009.* 2009 [cited 2009 July 22]; Available from: http://www.americanheart.org/presenter.jhtml?identifier=4475.

American Heart Association. *Cardiovascular disease statistics, 2006.* 2009 [cited 2009 July 22]; Available from: http://www.americanheart.org/presenter.jhtml?identifier=4478.

Antoni, M.H., *et al., The influence of bio-behavioural factors on tumour biology: pathways and mechanisms.* Nat Rev Cancer, 2006. **6**(3): p. 240-8.

Ashley, S.T. and W.S. Ashley, *Flood fatalities in the United States.* Journal of Applied Meteorology and Climatology, 2008. **47**(3): p. 805-818.

Attwood, S.W., *A Demographic-Analysis of Y-Neotricula Aperta (Gastropoda, Pomatiopsidae) Populations in Thailand and Southern Laos, in Relation to the Transmission of Schistosomiasis.* Journal of Molluscan Studies, 1995. **61**: p. 29-42.

Baccarelli, A., *et al., Exposure to particulate air pollution and risk of deep vein thrombosis.* Archives of Internal Medicine, 2008. **168**(9): p. 920-927.

Bacon, R.M., K.J. Kugeler, and P.S. Mead, *Surveillance for Lyme disease--United States, 1992-2006.* MMWR Surveill Summ, 2008. **57**(10): p. 1-9.

Balbus, J.M. and C. Malina, *Identifying vulnerable subpopulations for climate change health effects in the United States.* Journal of occupational and environmental medicine / American College of Occupational and Environmental Medicine, 2009. **51**(1): p. 33-37.

Ballester, F., J. Diaz, and J.M. Moreno, *[Climatic change and public health: scenarios after the coming into force of the Kyoto Protocol.].* Gac Sanit, 2006. **20 Suppl 1**: p. 160-74.

Balling, R.C. and R.S. Cerveny, *Compilation and discussion of trends in severe storms in the United States: Popular perception v. climate reality.* Natural Hazards, 2003. **29**(2): p. 103-112.

Barnett, A.G., *Temperature and cardiovascular deaths in the US elderly: changes over time.* Epidemiology, 2007. **18**(3): p. 369-72.

Bassil, K.L., *et al., Temporal and spatial variation of heat-related illness using 911 medical dispatch data.* Environmental Research, 2009. **109**(5): p. 600-606.

Bates, B., *et al., Climate change and water.* 2008, Intergovernmental Panel on Climate Change: Geneva. p. 210.

Batterman, S., *et al., Sustainable control of water-related infectious diseases: a review and proposal for interdisciplinary health-based systems research.* Environ Health Perspect, 2009. **117**(7): p. 1023-32.

Bedsworth, L., *Preparing for climate change: A perspective from local public health officers in California.* Environmental Health Perspectives, 2009. **117**(4): p. 617-623.

Beelen, R., *et al., Long-term exposure to traffic-related air pollution and lung cancer risk.* Epidemiology, 2008. **19**(5): p. 702-10.

Benson, V. and M.A. Marano, *Current estimates from the National Health Interview Survey, 1995.* Vital Health Stat 10, 1998. **190**. p. 1-428.

Black, H., *Unnatural disaster—Human factors in the Mississippi floods.* Environmental Health Perspectives, 2008. **116**(9): p. A390-+.

Black, P.H. and L.D. Garbutt, *Stress, inflammation and cardiovascular disease.* J Psychosom Res, 2002. **52**(1): p. 1-23.

Blanton, J.D., *et al., Rabies surveillance in the United States during 2007.* J Am Vet Med Assoc, 2008. **233**(6): p. 884-97.

Bocchi, E.A., *et al., Cardiomyopathy, adult valve disease and heart failure in South America.* Heart, 2009. **95**(3): p. 181-189.

Bolund, P. and S. Hunhammer, *Ecosystem services in urban areas.* Ecological Economics, 1999. **29**: p. 293-301.

Booth, S. and D. Zeller, *Mercury, food webs, and marine mammals: implications of diet and climate change for human health.* Environ Health Perspect, 2005. **113**(5): p. 521-6.

Bowker, G., *et al., The effects of roadside structures on the transport and dispersion of ultrafine particles from highways.* Atmospheric Environment, 2007. **41**: p. 8128-8139.

Boxall, A.B.A., *et al., Impacts of climate change on indirect human exposure to pathogens and chemicals from agriculture.* Environmental Health Perspectives, 2009. **117**(4): p. 508-514.

Brazel, A.J. and D. Quattrochi, *Urban Climates*, in *Encyclopedia of world climatology*, J.E. Oliver, Editor. 2005, Springer: Dordrecht, The Netherlands. p. xx, 854 p.

Brodie, E.C., *et al., Domoic acid causes reproductive failure in california sea lions (Zalophus californianus).* Marine Mammal Science, 2006. **22**(3): p. 700-707.

Bronstein, J., *et al., Meeting Report: Consensus Statement-Parkinson's Disease and the Environment: Collaborative on Health and the Environment and Parkinson's Action Network (CHE PAN) Conference 26-28 June 2007.* Environmental Health Perspectives, 2009. **117**(1): p. 117-121.

Brook, R.D., *Cardiovascular effects of air pollution.* Clinical Science, 2008. **115**(6): p. 175-187.

Brook, R.D., *et al., Air pollution and cardiovascular disease: a statement for healthcare professionals from the Expert Panel on Population and Prevention Science of the American Heart Association.* Circulation, 2004. **109**(21): p. 2655-71.

Brunkard, J.M., *et al., Dengue fever seroprevalence and risk factors, Texas-Mexico border, 2004.* Emerging Infectious Diseases, 2007. **13**(10): p. 1477-1483.

Bukowski, J.A., *Review of the epidemiological evidence relating toluene to reproductive outcomes.* Regul Toxicol Pharmacol, 2001. **33**(2): p. 147-56.

Burke, K.E. and H. Wei, *Synergistic damage by UVA radiation and pollutants.* Toxicol Ind Health, 2009. **25**(4-5): p. 219-24.

Burton, M. and M. Hicks, *Hurricane Katrina: Preliminary estimates of commercial and public sector damages.* 2005, Center for Business and Economic Research, Marshall University: Huntington, WV.

Bytomski, J.R. and D.L. Squire, *Heat illness in children.* Curr Sports Med Rep, 2003. **2**(6): p. 320-4.

Campbell-Lendrum, D., *et al., Health and climate change: a roadmap for applied research.* The Lancet, 2009. **373**(9676): p. 1663-1665.

Campbell-Lendrum, D., R. Woodruff, and WHO, *Climate Change: quantifying the health impactat national and local levels.* Environmental Burden of Disease Series, ed. A. Pruss-Ustun and C. Corvalan. 2007, Geneva: World Health Organization. 66.

Carcavallo, R.U., *Climatic factors related to Chagas disease transmission.* Memorias Do Instituto Oswaldo Cruz, 1999. **94**: p. 367-369.

Carod-Artal, F.J., *Strokes caused by infection in the tropics.* Revista De Neurologia, 2007. **44**(12): p. 755-763.

Carroll, J.F., *A note on the occurrence of the lone star tick, Amblyomma americanum in the greater Baltimore-Washington area.* Proc. of the Entomological Society of Washington, 2007. **109**(1): p. 253-256.

Carson, C., *et al., Declining vulnerability to temperature-related mortality in London over the 20th century.* Am J Epidemiol, 2006. **164**(1): p. 77-84.

Cassassa, G., *et al., Assessment of observed changes and responses in natural and managed systems.* 2007, Cambridge: Cambridge University Press.

CCSP, *Weather and Climate Extremes in a Changing Climate. Regions of Focus: North America, Hawaii, Caribbean, and U.S. Pacific Islands. A Report by the U.S. Climate Change Science Program and the Subcommittee on Global Change Research.*, T. Karl, *et al.*, Editors. 2008, Department of Commerce, NOAA's National Climatic Data Center: Washington, DC, USA. p. 164.

CDC. *Birth Defects.* 2009 [cited 2009 July 22]; Available from: http://www.cdc.gov/ncbddd/bd/.

Centers for Disease Control and Prevention. *Leading causes of death, 2006.* 2009 [cited 2009 July 22]; Available from: http://www.cdc.gov/nchs/FASTATS/lcod.htm.

Chico, T.J., P.W. Ingham, and D.C. Crossman, *Modeling cardiovascular disease in the zebrafish.* Trends Cardiovasc Med, 2008. **18**(4): p. 150-5.

Christensen, J.H., *et al., Regional Climate Projections*, in *Climate change 2007 : the physical science basis : contribution of Working Group I to the Fourth Assessment Report of the Intergovernmental Panel on Climate Change*, S. Solomon, Intergovernmental Panel on Climate Change., and Intergovernmental Panel on Climate Change. Working Group I., Editors. 2007, Cambridge University Press: Cambridge ; New York. p. 747-845.

Clougherty, J.E. and L.D. Kubzansky, *A framework for examining social stress and susceptibility to air pollution in respiratory health.* Environ Health Perspect, 2009. **117**(9): p. 1351-8.

Cohn, B.A., *et al., DDT and DDE exposure in mothers and time to pregnancy in daughters.* Lancet, 2003. **361**(9376): p. 2205-6.

Confalonieri, U., *et al., Human Health*, in *Climate Change 2007: Impacts, Adaptation and Vulnerability. Contribution of Working Group II to the Fourth Assessment Report of the Intergovernmental Panel on Climate Change*, M. Parry, *et al.*, Editors. 2007, Cambridge University Press: Cambridge. p. 391-431.

Constantin de Magny, G. and R.R. Colwell, *Cholera and climate: a demonstrated relationship.* Trans Am Clin Climatol Assoc, 2009. **120**: p. 119-28.

Correa-Villaseñor A., *et al., The Metropolitan Atlanta Congenital Defects Program: 35 years of birth defects surveillance at the Centers for Disease Control and Prevention.* Birth Defects Res A Clin Mol Teratol, 2003. **67**(9): p. 617-24.

Corvalán, C., *et al., Ecosystems and human well-being : health synthesis.* 2005, [Geneva, Switzerland]: World Health Organization. 53 p.

Corwin, D.L. and S.A. Bradford, *Environmental impacts and sustainability of degraded water reuse.* J Environ Qual, 2008. **37**(5 Suppl): p. S1-7.

Costello, A., *et al., Managing the health effects of climate change. Lancet and University College London Institute for Global Health Commission.* The Lancet, 2009. **373**(9676): p. 1693-1733.

Costello, S., *et al., Parkinson's disease and residential exposure to maneb and paraquat from agricultural applications in the central valley of California.* Am J Epidemiol, 2009. **169**(8): p. 919-26.

Cox, J. and M. Krajden, *Cardiovascular Manifestations of Lyme-Disease.* American Heart Journal, 1991. **122**(5): p. 1449-1455.

Craun, G.F. and R.L. Calderon, *Observational epidemiologic studies of endemic waterborne risks: cohort, case-control, time-series, and ecologic studies.* J Water Health, 2006. **4 Suppl 2**: p. 101-19.

Crowley, C., *The mental health needs of refugee children: a review of literature and implications for nurse practitioners.* J Am Acad Nurse Pract, 2009. **21**(6): p. 322-31.

Curriero, F.C., *et al., Temperature and mortality in 11 cities of the eastern United States.* Am J Epidemiol, 2002. **155**(1): p. 80-7.

Curriero, F.C., *et al.*, *The association between extreme precipitation and waterborne disease outbreaks in the United States, 1948-1994*. Am J Public Health, 2001. **91**(8): p. 1194-9.

D'Amato G. and L. Cecchi, *Effects of climate change on environmental factors in respiratory allergic diseases*. Clinical and Experimental Allergy, 2008. **38**(8): p. 1264-1274.

D'Amato G., *et al.*, *The role of outdoor air pollution and climatic changes on the rising trends in respiratory allergy*. Respiratory Medicine, 2001. **95**(7): p. 606-611.

Davido, A., *et al.*, *Risk factors for heat related death during the August 2003 heat wave in Paris, France, in patients evaluated at the emergency department of the Hopital Europeen Georges Pompidou*. Emerg Med J, 2006. **23**(7): p. 515-8.

Davis, R.E., *et al.*, *Changing heat-related mortality in the United States*. Environmental Health Perspectives, 2003. **111**(14): p. 1712-1718.

Davis, R.E., *et al.*, *Decadal changes in heat-related human mortality in the eastern United States*. Climate Research, 2002. **22**(2): p. 175-184.

Department of Homeland Security. *The First Year After Hurricane Katrina: What the Federal Government Did.* . 2009 [cited 2009 July 22]; Available from: www.dhs.gov/xfoia/archives/gc_1157649340100.shtm.

Deschenes, O. and M. Greenstone, *Climate Change, Mortality, and Adaptation: Evidence from Annual Fluctuations in Weather in the US*, in *Center for the Study of Energy Markets Paper*. 2007, Center for the Study of Energy Markets: Santa Barbara, CA. p. 61.

Diaz, J.H., *The influence of global warming on natural disasters and their public health outcomes*. Am J Disaster Med, 2007. **2**(1): p. 33-42.

Dong, S., *et al.*, *UVA-Induced DNA single-strand cleavage by 1-hydroxypyrene and formation of covalent adducts between DNA and 1-hydroxypyrene*. Chem Res Toxicol, 2000. **13**(7): p. 585-93.

Douglass, R.J., C.H. Calisher, and K.C. Bradley, *State-by-state incidences of hantavirus pulmonary syndrome in the United States, 1993-2004*. Vector Borne Zoonotic Dis, 2005. **5**(2): p. 189-92.

Dunglison, R., *On the influence of atmosphere and locality; change of air and climate; seasons; food; clothing; bathing; exercise; sleep; corporeal and intellectual pursuits, &c. &c. on human health; constituting elements of hygiene*. 1835, Philadelphia,: Carey, Lea & Blanchard. xi, [13]-514 p.

Dwight, R.H., *et al.*, *Health effects associated with recreational coastal water use: Urban versus rural California*. American Journal of Public Health, 2004. **94**(4): p. 565-567.

Dwight, R.H., *et al.*, *Association of urban runoff with coastal water quality in Orange County, California*. Water Environment Research, 2002. **74**(1): p. 82-90.

Easterling, D.R., *et al.*, *Climate extremes: Observations, modeling, and impacts*. Science, 2000. **289**(5487): p. 2068-2074.

Ebi, K., *et al.*, *Effects of Global Change on Human Health*, in *Analyses of the effects of global change on human health and welfare and human systems. A Report by the U.S. Climate Change Science Program and the Subcommittee on Global Change Research*, J. Gamble, *et al.*, Editors. 2008, USEPA: Washington, D. C.

Ebi, K.L., *et al.*, *Weather changes associated with hospitalizations for cardiovascular diseases and stroke in California, 1983-1998*. Int J Biometeorol, 2004. **49**(1): p. 48-58.

Ebi, K.L., *et al.*, *Climate suitability for stable malaria transmission in Zimbabwe under different climate change scenarios*. Climatic Change, 2005. **73**(3): p. 375-393.

Ebi, K.L., *et al.*, *Climate change and human health impacts in the United States: An update on the results of the U.S. National Assessment*. Environmental Health Perspectives, 2006. **114**(9): p. 1318-1324.

Eisenman, D.P., *et al.*, *Disaster planning and risk communication with vulnerable communities: lessons from Hurricane Katrina*. Am J Public Health, 2007. **97 Suppl 1**: p. S109-15.

Ellis, F.P., *Heat illness. I. Epidemiology*. Trans R Soc Trop Med Hyg, 1976. **70**(5-6): p. 402-11.

Ericksen, P.J., J.S.I. Ingram, and D.M. Liverman, *Food security and global environmental change: emerging challenges*. Environmental Science and Policy, 2009. **12**(4): p. 373-377.

Eskenazi, B., *et al.*, *Pesticide toxicity and the developing brain*. Basic Clin Pharmacol Toxicol, 2008. **102**(2): p. 228-36.

Estrada-Peña A., *Increasing habitat suitability in the United States for the tick that transmits Lyme disease: a remote sensing approach*. Environ Health Perspect, 2002. **110**(7): p. 635-40.

Faust, E., *Malaria Incidence in North America*, in *Malariology; a comprehensive survey of all aspects of this group of diseases from a global standpoint*, M.F. Boyd, Editor. 1949, Saunders: Philadelphia,. p. 2 v. (xxi, 1643 p.).

Feighner, B.H., *et al.*, *Reemergence of Plasmodium vivax malaria in the republic of Korea*. Emerg Infect Dis, 1998. **4**(2): p. 295-7.

Fleming, L.E., *et al.*, *Aerosolized red-tide toxins (brevetoxins) and asthma*. Chest, 2007. **131**(1): p. 187-194.

Flower, K.B., *et al.*, *Cancer risk and parental pesticide application in children of Agricultural Health Study participants*. Environ Health Perspect, 2004. **112**(5): p. 631-5.

Foley, D.H., *et al.*, *Geographic distribution and ecology of potential malaria vectors in the Republic of Korea*. J Med Entomol, 2009. **46**(3): p. 680-92.

Ford, T.E., *et al.*, *Using Satellite Images of Environmental Changes to Predict Infectious Disease Outbreaks*. Emerging Infectious Diseases, 2009. **15**(9): p. 1341-1346.

Fouillet, A., *et al.*, *Excess mortality related to the August 2003 heat wave in France*. International Archives of Occupational and Environmental Health, 2006. **80**(1): p. 16-24.

Fouillet, A., *et al.*, *Has the impact of heat waves on mortality changed in France since the European heat wave of summer 2003? A study of the 2006 heat wave*. Int J Epidemiol, 2008. **37**(2): p. 309-17.

Franzblau, A., *et al.*, *Residences with anomalous soil concentrations of dioxin-like compounds in two communities in Michigan, USA: A case study*. Chemosphere, 2009. **74**(3): p. 395-403.

Fritze, J.G., *et al.*, *Hope, despair and transformation: Climate change and the promotion of mental health and wellbeing*. Int J Ment Health Syst, 2008. **2**(1): p. 13.

Frumkin, H., L.D. Frank, and R. Jackson, *Urban sprawl and public health : designing, planning, and building for healthy communities*. 2004, Washington, DC: Island Press. xxi, 338 p.

Frumkin, H., *et al.*, *Climate change: The public health response*. American Journal of Public Health, 2008. **98**(3): p. 435-445.

Fthenakis, V., *Overview of potential hazards*, in *Practical handbook of photovoltaics : fundamentals and applications*, T. Markvart and L. Castañer, Editors. 2003, Elsevier Advanced Technology: New York.

Fthenakis, V.M., H.C. Kim, and E. Alsema, *Emissions from photovoltaic life cycles*. Environ Sci Technol, 2008. **42**(6): p. 2168-74.

Gage, K.L., *et al.*, *Climate and vectorborne diseases*. Am J Prev Med, 2008. **35**(5): p. 436-50.

Gamble, J.L. and K.L. Ebi, *Analyses of the effects of global change on human health and welfare and human systems : final report, synthesis and assessment product 4.6 : report by the U.S. Climate Change Science Program and the Subcommittee on Global Change Research*. 2008, Washington, D.C.: U.S. Climate Change Science Program. ix, 204 p.

Garland, C.F., *et al.*, *Vitamin D for cancer prevention: global perspective*. Ann Epidemiol, 2009. **19**(7): p. 468-83.

Gohlke, J.M., S.H. Hrynkow, and C.J. Portier, *Health, economy, and environment: Sustainable energy choices for a nation*. Environmental Health Perspectives, 2008. **116**(6): p. A236-A237.

Gong, H., *et al.*, *Cardiovascular effects of ozone exposure in human volunteers*. American Journal of Respiratory and Critical Care Medicine, 1998. **158**(2): p. 538-546.

Gosling, S.N., *et al.*, *Associations between elevated atmospheric temperature and human mortality: A critical review of the literature*. Climatic Change, 2009. **92**(3-4): p. 299-341.

Gosse, P., *Twenty-five years of research in hydroecology at the EDF research & development division*. Houille Blanche-Revue Internationale De L Eau, 1999. **54**(3-4): p. 95-102.

Green, R.S., *et al.*, *Residential exposure to traffic and spontaneous abortion*. Environ Health Perspect, 2009. **117**(12): p. 1939-44.

Greenough, G., *et al.*, *The potential impacts of climate variability and change on health impacts of extreme weather events in the United States*. Environmental Health Perspectives, 2001. **109**: p. 191-198.

Gregory, P.J., *et al.*, *Integrating pests and pathogens into the climate change/food security debate*. J Exp Bot, 2009. **60**(10): p. 2827-38.

Groisman, P.Y., *et al.*, *Changes in the probability of heavy precipitation: Important indicators of climatic change*. Climatic Change, 1999. **42**(1): p. 243-283.

Gustin, M.S. and K. Ladwig, *An assessment of the significance of mercury release from coal fly ash*. J Air Waste Manag Assoc, 2004. **54**(3): p. 320-30.

Haines, A., *et al.*, *Climate change and human health: impacts, vulnerability, and mitigation*. Lancet, 2006. **367**(9528): p. 2101-2109.

Haines, A., *et al.*, *Public health benefits of strategies to reduce greenhouse-gas emissions: overview and implications for policy makers*. Lancet, 2009.

Handal, A.J., *et al.*, *Neurobehavioral development in children with potential exposure to pesticides*. Epidemiology, 2007. **18**(3): p. 312-20.

Hardin, B.D., B.J. Kelman, and A. Saxon, *Adverse human health effects associated with molds in the indoor environment*. J Occup Environ Med, 2003. **45**(5): p. 470-8.

Hayhoe, K., *et al.*, *Emissions pathways, climate change, and impacts on California*. Proc Natl Acad Sci U S A, 2004. **101**(34): p. 12422-7.

Hayhoe, K., *et al.*, *Past and future changes in climate and hydrological indicators in the US Northeast*. Climate Dynamics, 2007. **28**(4): p. 381-407.

Heaney, C.D., *et al.*, *Contact with beach sand among beachgoers and risk of illness*. Am J Epidemiol, 2009. **170**(2): p. 164-72.

Henderson-Sellers, A., *et al.*, *Tropical cyclones and global climate change: A post-IPCC assessment*. Bulletin of the American Meteorological Society, 1998. **79**(1): p. 19-38.

Hendrie, H.C., *et al.*, *Alzheimer's disease, genes, and environment: The value of international studies*. Canadian Journal of Psychiatry-Revue Canadienne De Psychiatrie, 2004. **49**(2): p. 92-99.

Hill, J., *et al.*, *Environmental, economic, and energetic costs and benefits of biodiesel and ethanol biofuels*. Proc Natl Acad Sci U S A, 2006. **103**(30): p. 11206-10.

Hill, J., *et al.*, *Climate change and health costs of air emissions from biofuels and gasoline*. Proceedings of the National Academy of Sciences of the United States of America, 2009. **106**(6): p. 2077-2082.

Hollifield, M., *et al.*, *Measuring trauma and health status in refugees: a critical review*. Jama, 2002. **288**(5): p. 611-21.

Houghton, J.T. and Intergovernmental Panel on Climate Change. Working Group I., *Climate change 2001 : the scientific basis : contribution of Working Group I to the third assessment report of the Intergovernmental Panel on Climate Change*. 2001, Cambridge ; New York: Cambridge University Press. x, 881 p.

Hrudey, S.E., *et al.*, *A fatal waterborne disease epidemic in Walkerton, Ontario: comparison with other waterborne outbreaks in the developed world*. Water Science and Technology, 2003. **47**(3): p. 7-14.

Hunter, L.M., *Migration and environmental hazards*. Population and Environment, 2005. **26**(4): p. 273-302.

Institute of Medicine (U.S.). Committee on Achieving Sustainable Global Capacity for Surveillance and Response to Emerging Diseases of Zoonotic Origin. and G. Keusch, *Sustaining global surveillance and response to emerging zoonotic diseases*. 2009, Washington, DC: National Academies Press. xxv, 312 p.

Intergovernmental Panel on Climate Change. Working Group II., *Climate change 2007 : impacts, adaptation and vulnerability : contribution of Working Group II to the Fourth Assessment Report of the Intergovernmental Panel on Climate Change*. 2007, Cambridge: Cambridge University Press. ix, 976 p.

International Federation of Red Cross and Red Crescent Societies, *World Disaster Report 2009*, in *World Disaster Report*, L. Knight, Editor. 2009, International Federation of Red Cross and Red Crescent Societies: Geneva. p. 210.

Ito, S., T. Yokoyama, and K. Asakura, *Emissions of mercury and other trace elements from coal-fired power plants in Japan*. Sci Total Environ, 2006. **368**(1): p. 397-402.

Jentsch, A. and C. Beierkuhnlein, *Research frontiers in climate change: Effects of extreme meteorological events on ecosystems*. Comptes Rendus Geoscience, 2008. **340**(9-10): p. 621-628.

Jerrett, M., *et al.*, *Long-Term Ozone Exposure and Mortality*. New England Journal of Medicine, 2009. **360**(11): p. 1085-1095.

Jones, L., *et al.*, *Severe mental disorders in complex emergencies.* Lancet, 2009. **374**(9690): p. 654-61.

Kalkstein, L.S. and J.S. Greene, *An evaluation of climate/mortality relationships in large U.S. cities and the possible impacts of a climate change.* Environ Health Perspect, 1997. **105**(1): p. 84-93.

Kang, D., *et al.*, *Cancer incidence among pesticide applicators exposed to trifluralin in the Agricultural Health Study.* Environ Res, 2008. **107**(2): p. 271-6.

Kar, B.R., S.L. Rao, and B.A. Chandramouli, *Cognitive development in children with chronic protein energy malnutrition.* Behav Brain Funct, 2008. **4**: p. 31.

Karl, T., J. Melilo, and T. Peterson, *Global Climate ChangeImpacts in the United States.* 2009, New York: Cambridge University Press.

Karl, T., *et al.*, *Weather and climate extremes in a changing climate regions of focus: North America, Hawaii, Caribbean, and U.S. Pacific Islands,* in *Synthesis and assessment product 3.3.* 2008, U.S. Climate Change Science Program: Washington, DC. p. x, 162 p.

Kay, B.H., *et al.*, *Alphavirus infection in mosquitoes at the Ross River reservoir, north Queensland, 1990-1993.* Journal of the American Mosquito Control Association, 1996. **12**(3): p. 421-428.

Kessler, R.C., *et al.*, *Prevalence, severity, and comorbidity of 12-month DSM-IV disorders in the National Comorbidity Survey Replication.* Arch Gen Psychiatry, 2005. **62**(6): p. 617-27.

Kilbourne, E.M., *The spectrum of illness during heat waves.* Am J Prev Med, 1999. **16**(4): p. 359-60.

Kilbourne, E.M., *et al.*, *Risk factors for heatstroke. A case-control study.* JAMA, 1982. **247**(24): p. 3332-6.

Kim, Y.S., H.G. Choi, and K.W. Nam, *Seasonal variations of marine algal community in the vicinity of Uljin nuclear power plant, Korea.* Journal of Environmental Biology, 2008. **29**(4): p. 493-499.

Kirkpatrick, B., *et al.*, *Florida red tide and human health: a pilot beach conditions reporting system to minimize human exposure.* Sci Total Environ, 2008. **402**(1): p. 1-8.

Kistermann, T., *et al.*, *Microbial load of drinking water reservoir tributaries during extreme rainfall and runoff. .* Applied and Environmental Microbiology, 2002. **68**(5): p. 2188-2197.

Knutson, T. and R. Tuleya, *ropical cyclones and climate change: revisiting recent studies at GFDL,* in *Culture Extremes and Society.* 2008, Cambridge University Press: Cambridge.

Komatsu, K., *et al.*, *Increase in coccidioidomycosis - Arizona,1998-2001 (Reprinted from MMWR, vol 52, pg 109, 2003).* Journal of the American Medical Association, 2003. **289**(12): p. 1500-1502.

Kotermanski, S.E. and J.W. Johnson, *Mg2+ imparts NMDA receptor subtype selectivity to the Alzheimer's drug memantine.* J Neurosci, 2009. **29**(9): p. 2774-9.

Kovats, R.S. and S. Hajat, *Heat stress and public health: A critical review,* in *Annual Review of Public Health.* 2008. p. 41-55.

Kozma, C., *Neonatal toxicity and transient neurodevelopmental deficits following prenatal exposure to lithium: Another clinical report and a review of the literature.* Am J Med Genet A, 2005. **132**(4): p. 441-4.

Krewski, D., *et al.*, *Extended follow-up and spatial analysis of the American Cancer Society study linking particulate air pollution and mortality.* Res Rep Health Eff Inst, 2009(140): p. 5-114; discussion 115-36.

Kreyling, W.G., M. Semmler-Behnke, and W. Moller, *Ultrafine particle-lung interactions: does size matter?* J Aerosol Med, 2006. **19**(1): p. 74-83.

Krousel-Wood, M.A., *et al.*, *Medication adherence in older clinic patients with hypertension after Hurricane Katrina: Implications for clinical practice and disaster management.* American Journal of the Medical Sciences, 2008. **336**(2): p. 99-104.

Kunkel, K.E., *North American trends in extreme precipitation.* Natural Hazards, 2003. **29**(2): p. 291-305.

Kunkel, K.E., K. Andsager, and D.R. Easterling, *Long-term trends in extreme precipitation events over the conterminous United States and Canada.* Journal of Climate, 1999. **12**(8): p. 2515-2527.

Kysely, J., *et al.*, *Excess cardiovascular mortality associated with cold spells in the Czech Republic.* BMC Public Health, 2009 Jan 15;**9**:19.

Lake, I.R., *et al.*, *A re-evaluation of the impact of temperature and climate change on foodborne illness.* Epidemiol Infect, 2009. **137**, p. 1538–1547.

Landrigan, P.J., *et al.*, *The National Children's Study: a 21-year prospective study of 100,000 American children.* Pediatrics, 2006. **118**(5): p. 2173-86.

Law, D.C., *et al.*, *Maternal serum levels of polychlorinated biphenyls and 1,1-dichloro-2,2-bis(p-chlorophenyl) ethylene (DDE) and time to pregnancy.* Am J Epidemiol, 2005. **162**(6): p. 523-32.

Le Tertre, A., *et al.*, *Short-term effects of particulate air pollution on cardiovascular diseases in eight European cities.* J Epidemiol Community Health, 2002. **56**(10): p. 773-9.

Lefebvre, K.A., *et al.*, *Gene expression profiles in zebrafish brain after acute exposure to domoic acid at symptomatic and asymptomatic doses.* Toxicol Sci, 2009. **107**(1): p. 65-77.

LeGuenno, B., *Haemorrhagic fevers and ecological perturbations.* Arch Virol Suppl, 1997. **13**: p. 191-9.

Leiserowitz, A., E. Maibach, and C. Roser-Renouf, *Climate change in the American mind: Americans' climate change beliefs, attitudes, policy preferences, and actions.* 2009, Yale Project on Climate Change, Scool of Forestry and Environmental Sciences: New Haven, Connecticut. p. 56.

Leor, J., W.K. Poole, and R.A. Kloner, *Sudden cardiac death triggered by an earthquake.* New England Journal of Medicine, 1996. **334**(7): p. 413-419.

Longnecker, M.P., *et al.*, *Maternal serum level of 1,1-dichloro-2,2-bis(p-chlorophenyl)ethylene and risk of cryptorchidism, hypospadias, and polythelia among male offspring.* Am J Epidemiol, 2002. **155**(4): p. 313-22.

Longnecker, M.P., *et al.*, *Maternal serum level of the DDT metabolite DDE in relation to fetal loss in previous pregnancies.* Environ Res, 2005. **97**(2): p. 127-33.

Lovell, M.A., *A potential role for alterations of zinc and zinc transport proteins in the progression of Alzheimer's disease.* J Alzheimers Dis, 2009. **16**(3): p. 471-83.

Luber, G. and M. McGeehin, *Climate change and extreme heat events.* Am J Prev Med, 2008. **35**(5): p. 429-35.

Lynch, S.M., *et al.*, *Cancer incidence among pesticide applicators exposed to butylate in the Agricultural Health Study (AHS).* Environ Res, 2009. **109**(7): p. 860-8.

Mac Kenzie, W.R., *et al.*, *A massive outbreak in Milwaukee of cryptosporidium infection transmitted through the public water supply.* N Engl J Med, 1994. **331**(3): p. 161-7.

Macdonald, R.W., T. Harner, and J. Fyfe, *Recent climate change in the Arctic and its impact on contaminant pathways and interpretation of temporal trend data.* Sci Total Environ, 2005. **342**(1-3): p. 5-86.

Macdonald, R.W., *et al.*, *How will global climate change affect risks from long-range transport of persistent organic pollutants?* Human and Ecological Risk Assessment, 2003. **9**(3): p. 643-660.

Mahajan, R., *et al.*, *Fonofos exposure and cancer incidence in the agricultural health study.* Environ Health Perspect, 2006. **114**(12): p. 1838-42.

Maibach, E., C. Roser-Renouf, and A. Leiserowitz, *Global warming's six Americas 2009: An audience segmentation analysis.* 2009, George Mason University Center for Climate Change Communication: Washington, DC. p. 140.

Mann, J.K., *et al.*, *Air pollution and hospital admissions for ischemic heart disease in persons with congestive heart failure or arrhythmia.* Environmental Health Perspectives, 2002. **110**(12): p. 1247-1252.

Mannino, D.M., *et al.*, *Surveillance for asthma—United States, 1960-1995.* MMWR CDC Surveill Summ, 1998. **47**(1): p. 1-27.

Martin-Latry, K., *et al.*, *Psychotropic drugs use and risk of heat-related hospitalisation.* Eur Psychiatry, 2007. **22**(6): p. 335-8.

Massachusetts Institute of Technology., *The Future of nuclear power : an interdisciplinary MIT study.* 2003, [Boston MA]: MIT. x, 170 p.

Maszle, D.R., *et al.*, *Hydrological studies of schistosomiasis transport in Sichuan Province, China.* Science of the Total Environment, 1998. **216**(3): p. 193-203.

Mathers, C., *et al.*, *The global burden of disease : 2004 update.* 2008, Geneva, Switzerland: World Health Organization. vii, 146 p.

Mathers, J.C., *Early nutrition: Impact on epigenetics.* Nutrigenomics - Opportunities in Asia, 2007. **60**: p. 42-48.

Maucher, J.M. and J.S. Ramsdell, *Maternal-fetal transfer of domoic acid in rats at two gestational time points.* Environmental Health Perspectives, 2007. **115**(12): p. 1743-1746.

Mayeux, R., *Dissecting the relative influences of genes and the environment in Alzheimer's disease.* Annals of Neurology, 2004. **55**(2): p. 156-158.

McAloose, D. and A.L. Newton, *Wildlife cancer: a conservation perspective.* Nat Rev Cancer, 2009. **9**(7): p. 517-26.

McCormick, R.L., *The impact of biodiesel on pollutant emissions and public health.* Inhalation Toxicology, 2007. **19**(12): p. 1033-1039.

McGeehin, M.A. and M. Mirabelli, *The potential impacts of climate variability and change on temperature-related morbidity and mortality in the United States.* Environ Health Perspect, 2001. **109 Suppl 2**: p. 185-9.

McLaughlin, J.B., *et al.*, *Outbreak of Vibrio parahaemolyticus gastroenteritis associated with Alaskan oysters.* N Engl J Med, 2005. **353**(14): p. 1463-70.

McMichael, A.J., R.E. Woodruff, and S. Hales, *Climate change and human health: Present and future risks.* Lancet, 2006. **367**(9513): p. 859-869.

McPherson, E., *et al.*, *Quantifying urban forest structure, function, and value: the Chicago Urban Forest Climate Project. .* Urban Ecosystems, 1997. **1**: p. 49-61.

McQuiston, J.H., *et al.*, *National surveillance and the epidemiology of human Q fever in the United States, 1978-2004.* Am J Trop Med Hyg, 2006. **75**(1): p. 36-40.

Mead, P.S., *et al.*, *Food-related illness and death in the United States.* Emerg Infect Dis, 1999. **5**(5): p. 607-25.

Meehl, G.A. and C. Tebaldi, *More intense, more frequent, and longer lasting heat waves in the 21st century.* Science, 2004. **305**(5686): p. 994-7.

Meehl, G.A.a.S., T. F. and Collins, W. D. and Friedlingstein, A. T. and Gaye, A. T. and Gregory, J. M. and Kitoh, A. and Knutti, R. and Murphy, J. M. and Noda, A. and Raper, S. C. B. and Watterson, I. G. and Weaver, A. J. and Zhao, Z., *Global CLimate Projections,* in *Climate change 2007 : the physical science basis : contribution of Working Group I to the Fourth Assessment Report of the Intergovernmental Panel on Climate Change,* S. Solomon, Intergovernmental Panel on Climate Change., and Intergovernmental Panel on Climate Change. Working Group I., Editors. 2007, Cambridge University Press: Cambridge ; New York. p. 747-845.

Meinhardt, P.L., *Recognizing waterborne disease and the health effects of water contamination: a review of the challenges facing the medical community in the United States.* J Water Health, 2006. **4 Suppl 1**: p. 27-34.

Mendes, C.T., *et al.*, *Lithium reduces Gsk3b mRNA levels: implications for Alzheimer Disease.* Eur Arch Psychiatry Clin Neurosci, 2009. **259**(1): p. 16-22.

Merchandani, H., *et al.*, *Heat-Related Deaths - United-States, 1993 (Reprinted from Mmwr, Vol 42, 558-560, 1993).* ournal of the American Medical Association, 1993. **270**(7): p. 810-810.

Milan, D.J., *et al.*, *Drug-sensitized zebrafish screen identifies multiple genes, including GINS3, as regulators of myocardial repolarization.* Circulation, 2009. **120**(7): p. 553-9.

Miller, D.B. and J.P. O'Callaghan, *Do early-life insults contribute to the late-life development of Parkinson and Alzheimer diseases?* Metabolism, 2008. **57 Suppl 2**: p. S44-9.

Mills, D.M., *Climate Change, Extreme Weather Events, and US Health Impacts: What Can We Say?* Journal of Occupational and Environmental Medicine, 2009. **51**(1): p. 26-32.

Mills, E., *et al.*, *Prevalence of mental disorders and torture among Bhutanese refugees in Nepal: a systemic review and its policy implications.* Med Confl Surviv, 2008. **24**(1): p. 5-15.

Milly, P.C.D., K.A. Dunne, and A.V. Vecchia, *Global pattern of trends in streamflow and water availability in a changing climate.* Nature, 2005. **438**(7066): p. 347-350.

Moore, S.K., *et al.*, *Impacts of climate variability and future climate change on harmful algal blooms and human health.* Environmental Health: A Global Access Science Source, 2008. **7**(SUPPL. 2).

Morabito, M., *et al.*, *Relationships between weather and myocardial infarction: A biometeorological approach.* International Journal of Cardiology, 2005. **105**(3): p. 288-293.

Mos, L., *et al.*, *Chemical and biological pollution contribute to the immunological profiles of free-ranging harbor seals.* Environ Toxicol Chem, 2006. **25**(12): p. 3110-7.

Myers, N., *Environmental refugees: a growing phenomenon of the 21st century.* Philos Trans R Soc Lond B Biol Sci, 2002. **357**(1420): p. 609-13.

Naeem, F., *et al.*, *Psychiatric morbidity among Afghan refugees in Peshawar, Pakistan.* J Ayub Med Coll Abbottabad, 2005. **17**(2): p. 23-5.

Narukawa, T., et al., *Investigation on chemical species of arsenic, selenium and antimony in fly ash from coal fuel thermal power stations.* J Environ Monit, 2005. 7(12): p. 1342-8.

National Cancer Institute. *Lung Cancer.* 2009 [cited 2009 July 26]; Available from: http://www.cancer.gov/cancertopics/types/lung.

National Cancer Institute. *What is cancer?* 2009 [cited 2009 July 21]; Available from: http://www.cancer.gov/cancertopics/what-is-cancer.

National Research Council (U.S.). Committee on Ecological impacts of Climate Change., *Ecological impacts of climate change.* 2008, Washington, D.C.: National Academies Press. xii, 57 p.

National Research Council (U.S.). Committee On Health, E., And Other External Costs And, Benefits Of Energy Production And Consumption., and National Research Council (U.S.). Board on environmental studies and toxicology., *Hidden Costs of Energy: Unpriced Consequences of Energy Production and Use.* Board on Environmental Studies and Toxicology special report. 2009, Washington, D.C.: Board on Environmental Studies and Toxicology.

National Research Council (U.S.). Committee on Strategic Advice on the U.S. Climate Change Science Program., et al., *Restructuring federal climate research to meet the challenges of climate change.* 2009, Washington, D.C.: National Academies Press. xii, 254 p.

National Weather Service, *Summary of Natural Hazard Statistics for 2007 in the United States.* 2007: Washington.

Niemi, G., et al., *Rationale for a new generation of indicators for coastal waters.* Environmental Health Perspectives, 2004. 112(9): p. 979-986.

Nord, M., M. Andrews, and S. Carlson, *Hosehold food security in the United States, 2008*, E.R. Service, Editor. November, 2009, US Department of Agriculture: Washington, DC.

Nowak, D., D. Crane, and J. Stevens, *Air pollution removal by urban trees and shrubs in the United States.* Urban Forestry and Urban Greening, 2006. 4: p. 115-123.

Noyes, P.D., et al., *The toxicology of climate change: Environmental contaminants in a warming world.* Environment International, 2009. 35(6): p. 971-986.

NTP Report on Carcinogens. Rep Carcinog, 2005(11).

O'Neill MS., et al., *Air pollution and inflammation in type 2 diabetes: a mechanism for susceptibility.* Occupational and Environmental Medicine, 2007. 64(6): p. 373-379.

Orenstein, W.A., et al., *Immunizations in the United States: success, structure, and stress.* Health Aff (Millwood), 2005. 24(3): p. 599-610.

Paerl, H.W. and J. Huisman, *Climate. Blooms like it hot.* Science, 2008. 320(5872): p. 57-8.

Paik, Y.H., H.I. Ree, and J.C. Shim, *Malaria in Korea.* Jpn J Exp Med, 1988. 58(2): p. 55-66.

Papanikolaou, N.C., et al., *Lead toxicity update. A brief review.* Med Sci Monit, 2005. 11(10): p. RA329-36.

Park, S.K., et al., *Cancer incidence among paraquat exposed applicators in the agricultural health study: prospective cohort study.* Int J Occup Environ Health, 2009. 15(3): p. 274-81.

Patz, J., et al., *Health impact assessment of global climate change: Expanding on comparative risk assessment approaches for policy making,* in *Annual Review of Public Health.* 2008. p. 27-39.

Patz, J.A., et al., *Impact of regional climate change on human health.* Nature, 2005. 438(7066): p. 310-7.

Patz, J.A., et al., *Climate change and waterborne disease risk in the Great Lakes region of the U.S.* Am J Prev Med, 2008. 35(5): p. 451-8.

Pavlin, B.I., L.M. Schloegel, and P. Daszak, *Risk of importing zoonotic diseases through wildlife trade, United States.* Emerg Infect Dis, 2009. 15(11): p. 1721-6.

Peters, A., et al., *Increased particulate air pollution and the triggering of myocardial infarction.* Circulation, 2001. 103(23): p. 2810-2815.

Petri, W.A., Jr., *America in the world: 100 years of tropical medicine and hygiene.* Am J Trop Med Hyg, 2004. 71(1): p. 2-16.

Piver, W.T., et al., *Temperature and air pollution as risk factors for heat stroke in Tokyo, July and August 1980-1995.* Environ Health Perspect, 1999. 107(11): p. 911-6.

Planton, S., *Global warming and El Nino: a review of the current knowledge.* Medecine Et Maladies Infectieuses, 1999. 29(5): p. 267-276.

Pope, C.A., 3rd, et al., *Lung cancer, cardiopulmonary mortality, and long-term exposure to fine particulate air pollution.* JAMA, 2002. 287(9): p. 1132-41.

Pope, C.A. and D.W. Dockery, *Health effects of fine particulate air pollution: Lines that connect.* Journal of the Air & Waste Management Association, 2006. 56(6): p. 709-742.

Potapova, M. and P. Snoeijs, *The natural life cycle in wild populations of Diatoma moniliformis (Bacillariophyceae) and its disruption in an aberrant environment.* Journal of Phycology, 1997. 33(6): p. 924-937.

Pradat, P., et al., *First trimester exposure to corticosteroids and oral clefts.* Birth Defects Res A Clin Mol Teratol, 2003. 67(12): p. 968-70.

Prüss-Üstün, A., C. Corvalán, and World Health Organization., *Preventing disease through healthy environments : towards an estimate of the environmental burden of disease.* 2006, Geneva, Switzerland: World Health Organization. 104 p.

Qian Z, et al., *High temperatures enhanced acute mortality effects of ambient particle pollution in the "Oven" city of Wuhan, China.* Environmental Health Perspectives, 2008. 116(9): p. 1172-1178.

Quinn, J.F., et al., *Copper in Alzheimer's disease: too much or too little?* Expert Rev Neurother, 2009. 9(5): p. 631-7.

Ramsdell, J.S. and T.S. Zabka, *In utero domoic acid toxicity: a fetal basis to adult disease in the California sea lion (Zalophus californianus).* Marine Drugs, 2008. 6(2): p. 262-90.

Rappaport, E.N., et al., *Advances and Challenges at the National Hurricane Center.* Weather and Forecasting, 2009. 24(2): p. 395-419.

Ree, H.I., *Unstable vivax malaria in Korea.* Korean J Parasitol, 2000. 38(3): p. 119-38.

Reiter, P., et al., *Texas lifestyle limits transmission of dengue virus.* Emerging Infectious Diseases, 2003. 9(1): p. 86-89.

Ren, C., et al., *Ozone modifies associations between temperature and cardiovascular mortality: analysis of the NMMAPS data.* Occupational and Environmental Medicine, 2008. 65(4): p. 255-260.

Ribas-Fitó N., et al., *Prenatal exposure to 1,1-dichloro-2,2-bis (p-chlorophenyl)ethylene (p,p'-DDE) in relation to child growth.* Int J Epidemiol, 2006. 35(4): p. 853-8.

Roeleveld, N. and R. Bretveld, *The impact of pesticides on male fertility.* Curr Opin Obstet Gynecol, 2008. 20(3): p. 229-33.

Rogan, W.J. and N.B. Ragan, *Some evidence of effects of environmental chemicals on the endocrine system in children.* Int J Hyg Environ Health, 2007. 210(5): p. 659-67.

Rogers, C.A., et al., *Interaction of the onset of spring and elevated atmospheric CO2 on ragweed (Ambrosia artemisiifolia L.) pollen production.* Environmental Health Perspectives, 2006. 114(6): p. 865-869.

Rogers, D.J. and S.E. Randolph, *The global spread of malaria in a future, warmer world.* Science, 2000. 289(5485): p. 1763-6.

Rosas, L.G. and B. Eskenazi, *Pesticides and child neurodevelopment.* Curr Opin Pediatr, 2008. 20(2): p. 191-7.

Rudowitz, R., D. Rowland, and A. Shartzer, *Health care in New Orleans before and after Hurricane Katrina.* Health Aff (Millwood), 2006. 25(5): p. w393-406.

Ruidavets, J.B., et al., *Ozone air pollution is associated with acute myocardial infarction.* Circulation, 2005. 111(5): p. 563-569.

Rusiecki, J.A., et al., *Cancer incidence among pesticide applicators exposed to permethrin in the Agricultural Health Study.* Environ Health Perspect, 2009. 117(4): p. 581-6.

Samoli, E., et al., *Acute Effects of Ambient Particulate Matter on Mortality in Europe and North America: Results from the APHENA Study.* Environmental Health Perspectives, 2008. 116(11): p. 1480-1486.

Sandifer, P., et al., *Interagency oceans and human health research implementation plan: a prescription for the future.* 2007, Interagency Working Group on Harmful Algal Blooms, Hypoxia and Human Health of the Joint Subcommittee on Ocean Science and Technology: Washington, DC, USA.

Schwartz, J., J.M. Samet, and J.A. Patz, *Hospital admissions for heart disease - The effects of temperature and humidity.* Epidemiology, 2004. 15(6): p. 755-761.

Scoville, A., *Epidemic typhus fever in Japan and Korea,* in *Rickettsial diseases of man; a symposium,* F.R. Moulton, Editor. 1948, American Association for the Advancement of Science.: Washington, D.C,. p. 247 p.

Semenza, J.C. and B. Menne, *Climate change and infectious diseases in Europe.* Lancet Infectious Diseases, 2009. 9(6): p. 365-375.

Senhorst, H.A.J. and J.J.G. Zwolsman, *Climate change and effects on water quality: a first impression.* Water Science and Technology, 2005. 51(5): p. 53-59.

Shea, K.M., et al., *Climate change and allergic disease.* Journal of Allergy and Clinical Immunology, 2008. 122(3): p. 443-453.

Sheridan, S.C., A.J. Kalkstein, and L.S. Kalkstein, *Trends in heat-related mortality in the United States, 1975-2004.* Natural Hazards, 2009. 50(1): p. 145-160.

Shultz, A., et al., *Cholera Outbreak in Kenyan Refugee Camp: Risk Factors for Illness and Importance of Sanitation.* American Journal of Tropical Medicine and Hygiene, 2009. 80(4): p. 640-645.

Sidley, P., *Floods in southern Africa result in cholera outbreak and displacement.* BMJ, 2008. 336(7642): p. 471.

Silove, D. and Z. Steel, *Understanding community psychosocial needs after disasters: implications for mental health services.* J Postgrad Med, 2006. 52(2): p. 121-5.

Sleijffers, A., et al., *Ultraviolet light and resistance to infectious diseases.* J Immunotoxicol, 2004. 1(1): p. 3-14.

Smith, D.H., et al., *A national estimate of the economic costs of asthma.* Am J Respir Crit Care Med, 1997. 156(3 Pt 1): p. 787-93.

Smith, K.R., et al., *Public health benefits of strategies to reduce greenhouse-gas emissions: health implications of short-lived greenhouse pollutants.* Lancet, 2009.

Smolinski, M.S., et al., *Microbial threats to health : emergence, detection, and response.* 2003, Washington, D.C.: National Academies Press. xxviii, 367 p.

Sokurenko, E.V., R. Gomulkiewicz, and D.E. Dykhuizen, *Source-sink dynamics of virulence evolution.* Nat Rev Microbiol, 2006. 4(7): p. 548-55.

Steenland, K., et al., *Recent trends in Alzheimer disease mortality in the United States, 1999 to 2004.* Alzheimer Dis Assoc Disord, 2009. 23(2): p. 165-70.

Stein, J., et al., *In harm's way: toxic threats to child development.* J Dev Behav Pediatr, 2002. 23(1 Suppl): p. S13-22.

Stewart, J.R., et al., *The coastal environment and human health: microbial indicators, pathogens, sentinels and reservoirs.* Environ Health, 2008. 7 Suppl 2: p. S3.

Stitt, M., *Rising Co2 Levels and Their Potential Significance for Carbon Flow in Photosynthetic Cells.* Plant Cell and Environment, 1991. 14(8): p. 741-762.

Strickman, D., S.P. Frances, and M. Debboun, *Prevention of bug bites, stings, and disease.* 2009, Oxford ; New York: Oxford University Press. xviii, 323 p., [8] p. of plates.

Strickman, D. and P. Kittayapong, *Dengue and its vectors in Thailand: Calculated transmission risk from total pupal counts of Aedes aegypti and association of wing-length measurements with aspects of the larval habitat.* American Journal of Tropical Medicine and Hygiene, 2003. 68(2): p. 209-217.

Study of Critical Environmental Problems. and Massachusetts Institute of Technology., *Man's impact on the global environment; assessment and recommendations for action; report or the Study of Critical Environmental Problems (SCEP).* 1970, Cambridge, Mass.,: MIT Press. xxii, 319 p.

Sur, D., et al., *Severe cholera outbreak following floods in a northern district of West Bengal.* Indian J Med Res, 2000. 112: p. 178-82.

Surwit, R.S., et al., *Stress management improves long-term glycemic control in type 2 diabetes.* Diabetes Care, 2002. 25(1): p. 30-4.

Suzuki, S., et al., *Hanshin-Awaji earthquake as a trigger for acute myocardial infarction.* American Heart Journal, 1997. 134(5): p. 974-977.

Swanson, K.J., M.C. Madden, and A.J. Ghio, *Biodiesel exhaust: The need for health effects research.* Environmental Health Perspectives, 2007. 115(4): p. 496-499.

Tapsell, S.M., et al., *Vulnerability to flooding: health and social dimensions.* Philos Transact A Math Phys Eng Sci, 2002. **360**(1796): p. 1511-25.

The CNA Corporation, *National Security and the Threat of Climate Change.* 2007: p. 68.

Thomson, M.C. and S.J. Connor, *The development of malaria early warning systems for Africa.* Trends in Parasitology, 2001. **17**(9): p. 438-445.

Tofail, F., et al., *Effect of Arsenic Exposure during Pregnancy on Infant Development at 7 Months in Rural Matlab, Bangladesh.* Environmental Health Perspectives, 2009. **117**(2): p. 288-293.

Tolba, O., et al., *Survival of epidemic strains of healthcare (HA-MRSA) and community-associated (CA-MRSA) meticillin-resistant Staphylococcus aureus (MRSA) in river-, sea- and swimming pool water.* Int J Hyg Environ Health, 2008. **211**(3-4): p. 398-402.

Toyooka, T., et al., *Coexposure to benzo[a]pyrene and UVA induces DNA damage: first proof of double-strand breaks in a cell-free system.* Environ Mol Mutagen, 2006. **47**(1): p. 38-47.

Trenberth, K.E., et al., *The changing character of precipitation.* Bulletin of the American Meteorological Society, 2003. **84**(9): p. 1205-+.

Tromel, S. and C.D. Schonwiese, *Probability change of extreme precipitation observed from 1901 to 2000 in Germany.* Theoretical and Applied Climatology, 2007. **87**(1-4): p. 29-39.

Tromp, T.K., et al., *Potential environmental impact of a hydrogen economy on the stratosphere.* Science, 2003. **300**(5626): p. 1740-2.

Tucker, M.A., *Melanoma epidemiology.* Hematol Oncol Clin North Am, 2009. **23**(3): p. 383-95, vii.

United Nations Department of Economic and Social Affairs Population Division *World Urbanization Prospects: The 2005 Revision,* P.D. United Nations Department of Economic and Social Affairs, Editor. 2006, United Nations Department of Economic and Social Affairs, Population Division: Geneva.

United States. Congress. Senate. Committee on Commerce Science and Transportation., *Oceans and Human Health Act: report of the Committee on Commerce, Science, and Transportation on S. 1218.* 2003, Washington: U.S. G.P.O. ii. 8 p.

US Environmental Protection Agency, *Report to Congress: impacts and control of CSOs and SSOs. Office of Wastewater Management.* 2004, US Environmental Protection Agency,: Washington, DC.

US Food and Drug Administration, *Quantitative risk assessment on the public health impact of pathogenic Vibrio parahaemolyticus in raw oysters.* 2005.

Uysal, N. and R.M. Schapira, *Effects of ozone on lung function and lung diseases.* Curr Opin Pulm Med, 2003. **9**(2): p. 144-50.

van der Leun, J.C., R.D. Piacentini, and F.R. de Gruijl, *Climate change and human skin cancer.* Photochem Photobiol Sci, 2008. **7**(6): p. 730-3.

Vandentorren, S., et al., *Mortality in 13 French cities during the August 2003 heat wave.* Am J Public Health, 2004. **94**(9): p. 1518-20.

Vasconcelos, C.H. and E. Novo, *Influence of recipitation, deforestation and Tucurui reservoir operation on malaria incidence rates in southeast Para, Brazil.* Igarss 2003: Ieee International Geoscience and Remote Sensing Symposium, Vols I - Vii, Proceedings, 2003: p. 4567-4569

Verger, P., et al., *Assessment of exposure to a flood disaster in a mental-health study.* Journal of Exposure Analysis and Environmental Epidemiology, 2003. **13**(6): p. 436-442.

Vose, R.S., et al., *Climate - Impact of land-use change on climate.* Nature, 2004. **427**(6971): p. 213-214.

Vugla, D.J., et al., *Increase in Coccidioidomycosis-California, 2000-2007 (Reprinted from MMWR, vol 58, pg 105-109, 2009).* Journal of the American Medical Association, 2009. **301**(17): p. 1760-1762.

Wadhwa, P.D., et al., *Developmental origins of health and disease: brief history of the approach and current focus on epigenetic mechanisms.* Semin Reprod Med, 2009. **27**(5): p. 358-68.

Wainwright, S., S. Buchanan, and H. Mainzer, *Cardiovascular Mortality - the Hidden Peril of Heat Waves.* American Journal of Epidemiology, 1994. **139**(11): p. S49-S49.

Wan, S.Q., et al., *Response of an allergenic species Ambrosia psilostachya (Asteraceae), to experimental warming and clipping: Implications for public health.* American Journal of Botany, 2002. **89**(11): p. 1843-1846.

Wang, D.Z., *Neurotoxins from marine dinoflagellates: a brief review.* Marine Drugs, 2008. **6**(2): p. 349-71.

Wang, W., et al., *Detecting changes in extreme precipitation and extreme streamflow in the Dongjiang River Basin in southern China.* Hydrology and Earth System Sciences, 2008. **12**(1): p. 207-221.

Watanabe, H., et al., *Impact of earthquakes on Takotsubo cardiomyopathy.* Journal of the American Medical Association, 2005. **294**(3): p. 305-307.

Weisler, R.H., J.G.t. Barbee, and M.H. Townsend, *Mental health and recovery in the Gulf Coast after Hurricanes Katrina and Rita.* JAMA, 2006. **296**(5): p. 585-8.

Weiss, K.B., P.J. Gergen, and T.A. Hodgson, *An economic evaluation of asthma in the United States.* N Engl J Med, 1992. **326**(13): p. 862-6.

White, C.M., et al., *Sequestration of carbon dioxide in coal with enhanced coalbed methane recovery - A review.* Energy & Fuels, 2005. **19**(3): p. 659-724.

White, P.C., Jr., *Murine Typhus in Fulton County, Georgia.* Mil Med, 1965. **130**: p. 386-8.

WHO, *Monitoring Antimalarial Drug Resistance.* 2002, Geneva: World Health Organization. xx, 190 p.

WHO. Global Malaria Programme., *World malaria report, 2008.* 2008, Geneva: World Health Organization. xx, 190 p.

Wilby, R., M. Hedger, and H. Orr, *Climate change impacts and adaptation: A science agenda for the Environment Agency of England and Wales.* Weather, Volume 60, Issue 7. p. 206-211.

Wilkinson, P., et al., *Public health benefits of strategies to reduce greenhouse-gas emissions: household energy.* Lancet, 2009. **374**(9705): p. 1917-29.

Wilmoth, J.M. and C.F. Longino, *Demographic trends that will shape US policy in the twenty-first century.* Research on Aging, 2006. **28**(3): p. 269-288.

Woodcock, J., et al., *Public health benefits of strategies to reduce greenhouse-gas emissions: urban land transport.* Lancet, 2009. **374**(9705): p. 1930-43.

Ye, F., et al., *Effects of temperature and air pollutants on cardiovascular and respiratory diseases for males and females older than 65 years of age in Tokyo, July and August 1980-1995.* Environ Health Perspect, 2001. **109**(4): p. 355-9.

Yoder, J., et al., *Surveillance for waterborne disease and outbreaks associated with drinking water and water not intended for drinking--United States, 2005-2006.* MMWR Surveill Summ, 2008. **57**(9): p. 39-62.

Yohannes, M., et al., *Can source reduction of mosquito larval habitat reduce malaria transmission in Tigray, Ethiopia?* Tropical Medicine & International Health, 2005. **10**(12): p. 1274-1285.

Yoshida, Y., *Development of air conditioning technologies to reduce CO2 emissions in the commercial sector.* Carbon Balance Manag, 2006. **1**: p. 12.

Zanobetti, A., et al., *The temporal pattern of respiratory and heart disease mortality in response to air pollution.* Environ Health Perspect, 2003. **111**(9): p. 1188-93.

Zhou, G., et al., *Climate variability and malaria epidemics in the highlands of East Africa.* Trends Parasitol, 2005. **21**(2): p. 54-6.

Ziska, L.H., et al., *Alterations in the production and concentration of selected alkaloids as a function of rising atmospheric carbon dioxide and air temperature: implications for ethno-pharmacology.* Global Change Biology, 2005. **11**(10): p. 1798-1807.

PHOTOGRAPHY CREDITS

COVER:
The cover image is a composite of an EVEREST (Exploratory Visualization Environment for REsearch in Science and Technology) map of the United States and a group of intertwined hands, symbolizing the need to work together to address the health effects of climate change. Image courtesy of the National Center for Computational Sciences, Oak Ridge National Laboratory

PAGE 8:
Top Right—© Jim Reed/Science Faction/Corbis
Bottom—© Karen Kasmauski/Corbis

PAGE 12:
Top Right—© Jim Reed/Science Faction/Corbis
Bottom—© Bob Sacha/Corbis

PAGE 16:
Bottom—© Simon Jarratt/Corbis

PAGE 20:
Bottom—© Scott Houston/Sygma/Corbis

PAGE 24:
Bottom—© David Gubernick/AgStock Images/Corbis

PAGE 25:
http://www.nwfsc.noaa.gov/publications/newsletters/fishmatters/highlights2004/highlights2004.cfm

PAGE 25:
© David Gubernick/AgStock Images/Corbis

PAGE 28:
Bottom—© Corbis

PAGE 33:
Frank Hadley Collins, Director, Center for Global Health and Infectious Diseases, University of Notre Dame

PAGE 36:
Top Right—© AP Photos/Stephan Savoia
Bottom— Marty Bahamonde/FEMA

PAGE 40:
Top Right—Vera Trainer/NOAA
Bottom—© Brooks Kraft/Corbis

PAGE 44:
Top Right and Bottom—© Karen Kasmauski/Science Faction/Corbis

PAGE 45:
© Karen Kasmauski/Science Faction/Corbis

PAGE 50:
Top Right—© Dennis Kunkel Microscopy, Inc.

PAGE 51:
EPA— http://www.epa.gov/glnpo/atlas/index.html

PAGE 56:
Bottom—© Jerry McCrea/The Star Ledger

ACKNOWLEDGMENTS

We would like to thank our colleagues who reviewed versions of the document, contributed examples and information, and otherwise supported this process.

EPA: Rona Birnbaum, Carl Mazza, PhD, Al McGartland, PhD, Bruce Rodan, MD, the EPA Climate Change and Health *ad hoc* working group, the Science Policy Council Steering Committee, the EPA Climate Change Science Program Synthesis 4.6 Reviewers, the Office of Air and Radiation, the Office of Research and Development, and the Office of Policy, Economics, and Innovation.

NIEHS: John Balbus, MD, MPH; Tonya Stonham

Brogan & Partners: Joseph W. Tart (design and layout), Mary Edbrooke (typography and layout)

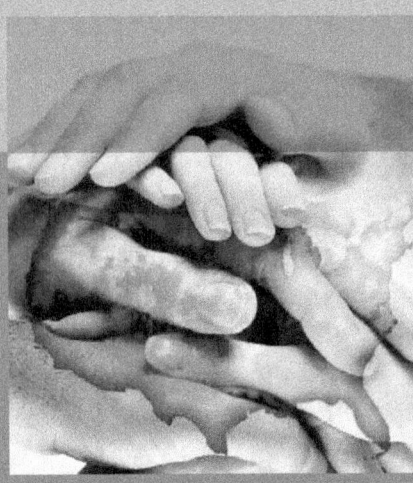

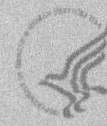 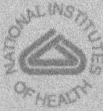 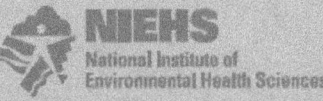

NIEHS
National Institute of
Environmental Health Sciences

ehp | ENVIRONMENTAL HEALTH PERSPECTIVES

PUBLISHED BY: *Environmental Health Perspectives and*
the National Institute of Environmental Health Sciences

PRINTED ON: NEW LEAF SAKURA | 100% DE-INKED RECYCLED | 50% POST CONSUMER WASTE
PROCESSED CHLORINE FREE GREEN E® CERTIFIED | ANCIENT FOREST FRIENDLY